Experience, Evidence and Everyday Practice

Creating systems for delivering effective health care

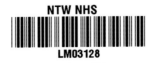

Experience, Evidence and Everyday Practice

Creating systems for delivering effective health care

Michael Dunning, Gerrard Abi-Aad, David Gilbert, Hayley Hutton and Clare Brown

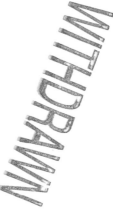

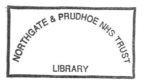
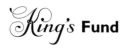

King's Fund

Published by
King's Fund Publishing
11–13 Cavendish Square
London W1M 0AN

© King's Fund 1999

First published 1999   Reprinted 1999

ISBN 1 85717 239 6

A CIP catalogue record for this book is available from the British Library

Available from:
King's Fund Bookshop
11–13 Cavendish Square
LONDON
W1M 0AN

Tel: 0171 307 2591
Fax: 0171 307 2801

Printed and bound in Great Britain

Cover illustration by Minuche Mazumdar Farrar

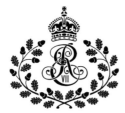

Contents

Preface   *vii*

Summary   *viii*

Introduction   *xi*

1   Setting the context   1

2   Building on the evidence, learning from experience   7

3   The local projects   35

    The care and treatment of cardiac patients   37
        Lambeth, Southwark and Lewisham and King's Healthcare:
        cardiac rehabilitation   37
        North Derbyshire: congestive cardiac failure   41
        South Tyneside: the management of stable angina   46
    The prevention and management of stroke   53
        Barnet: hypertension in the elderly   53
        Gloucestershire Royal: the management of stroke patients   56
    The care and treatment of people with mental health problems   62
        Wirral: family support in schizophrenia   62
    The eradication of *H. pylori* in the management of dyspepsia   67
        Bradford   69
        Bromley   73
        Walsall   78
    The management of continence   83
        Dudley   83
        Wigan and Bolton   88
    The care and treatment of patients predominantly in primary care   93
        Dorset: menorrhagia   93
        Royal Berkshire: leg ulcers   98
        Southern Derbyshire: back pain   102
    The care of patients in hospital   106
        Chase Farm: pressure sores   106
        Oxfordshire: post-operative pain control   110

Appendix: Contacts for the 16 local projects   117

Preface

Over the last three years an extensive network of people involved in 16 projects across England have been working with us to help us – as the main part of the Promoting Action on Clinical Effectiveness (PACE) programme – understand how to implement change in clinical practice. They have shown that change can be achieved if there is sound evidence on which to base the work, and if a project approach to managing implementation is adopted.

It is, however, a costly and messy process. It requires significant resources, time, people and materials to drive the work on. Moreover, it is not a logical, linear task with clearly defined stages to the work, but rather a group of complex, inter-related tasks which require skill and dexterity to manage to a satisfactory conclusion. The key message from research – that a multi-faceted approach using a range of techniques can be successful – has been confirmed. But the continuing use of projects running alongside local systems to implement change may not be sustainable in the long term. As the concept of clinical governance goes forward, organisations must find ways to develop a systems approach to securing improvements in the quality of clinical practice. The PACE experience offers many valuable lessons that will be relevant to that work.

Some projects have made more progress than others – both in the changes they have been able to achieve in the time available and in how they have been able to define and build on the learning from their work. The timescale for the programme and the nature of information systems in the NHS have limited the extent to which we can, at this stage, report on the impact of the local projects. We hope that ways can be found to revisit the projects later to quantify the longer-term impact of their work. Such information could add significantly to the body of knowledge about implementing change.

Throughout the programme, we have encouraged openness and honesty: openness about progress and honesty about mistakes and problems. This has enabled us to be clear about 'what works'. The programme has been characterised by the determined and skilled efforts of all those involved in the local projects who have worked hard to make a success of PACE. This report is a tribute to their efforts.

Michael Dunning
Gerrard Abi-Aad
David Gilbert
Hayley Hutton
Clare Brown

December 1998

Summary

Practical experience gained by those involved in the 16 PACE projects and the emerging research evidence about changing clinical practice and developing organisations provide the basis for this report. It draws together the essential attributes of the successful management of implementation initiatives – awareness of the emerging *evidence* about changing clinical behaviour and organisational development, the value of *experience* of managing change in the Health Service and the need for local *knowledge* and understanding of organisational structures and relationships.

The PACE experience has confirmed that a multi-faceted approach – using a range of techniques – can be successful, but implementation:

- *is a messy business*, requiring facilitation, flexibility and project leaders able to coax, cajole and drive the work forward
- *is not a linear task*, but rather a group of complex inter-related tasks
- *takes time*, usually far longer than expected
- *is expensive*, requiring lots of commitment if success is to be achieved.

Overall though, the experience shows this effort to be worthwhile. Improvements to the care and treatment of patients have been achieved, and the local projects have enabled many people to develop new skills and working relationships. The 'cost' is thus an investment with the initial steep learning curve becoming easier. Many of the local projects have been catalysts for a range of related activities, such as the development of local implementation programmes covering a range of clinical conditions.

Ten essential tasks have been identified which, when used together as components of an overall implementation programme, can lead to success. These tasks need to be managed into a coherent whole, with those leading the work having to *link* and *balance* efforts between parallel activities:

- **choosing where to start** and ensuring that there is support locally for the proposal. Action is required on: establishing criteria to choose the topic, assessing current practice, assembling evidence and determining local priorities
- **engaging clinicians** and securing their support for the proposed initiative – by understanding the local context, identifying local clinical leaders and recognising barriers to change
- **involving patients** means being clear about *why* patients need to be involved and *how* to do so

- *defining local standards* involves agreeing, locally, the intended standard of practice. Action is required on how standards will be presented, creating local guidelines and demonstrating the benefits of change
- *keeping in touch* with those affected as the work is taken forward. Communications must be taken seriously with clarity about the messages, the role of the messenger and existing communications systems
- *securing change* is the core of the work and involves a range of activities. It will mean considering an incremental approach, enlisting the support of clinical leaders, supporting the development of teams, providing education and training, developing audit tools and providing support to make change happen
- *providing services* to match the proposed changes to clinical practice. An assessment of the service and resource consequences of the initiative will be required and ensuring a link with planning and budgeting timetables
- *measuring impact* to demonstrate achievement: being clear about what to measure and identifying ways to capture relevant data
- *sustaining change* to ensure that changes become routine practice. Action will be required to ensure the supply of new documentation, creating reminder systems, providing induction training and promoting achievements
- *learning lessons* by managing the work as a learning experience and ensuring that similar, subsequent activities build on the successes (and failures) of the work.

Successful implementation requires a sound project management approach. Clarity is needed about who will lead the work – preferably a locally respected and knowledgeable senior clinician – and who will undertake day-to-day co-ordination. Effective teamworking is important, calling for a wide range of skills and contributions. The roles of clinicians and managers within the initiative will require careful consideration: implementing change in clinical practice is not solely a clinical issue.

However, because of the costs involved, reliance on discrete projects not embedded into local systems, to deliver improvements in practice will not be sustainable in the long-term. This will be emphasised if the work of the National Institute for Clinical Excellence matches the Government's aims – with an extensive programme of work, through National Service Frameworks, etc.

Effective local arrangements for clinical governance will require organisations to put in place systems to assure the delivery of high quality health care. The PACE experience suggests that local organisations will need to put in place five linked systems. First, to enable clinical staff to review, routinely, the quality of current practice. Second, to ensure that standards for care can be established. Third, to ensure that patients are at the centre of work which develops and monitors local standards.

Fourth, to ensure that the implementation is managed effectively. Fifth, to support the development of individuals and clinical teams through a systematic approach to education and training.

Senior leadership should ensure that these systems are effectively inter-connected. A management style which involve all staff and encourages open discussions about, and learning from, problems will be essential. Systems management will become as important as performance management.

Introduction

Between 1995 and 1998, the Promoting Action on Clinical Effectiveness (PACE) programme provided a national focus to support the development of knowledge and understanding about how to implement evidence-based practice. The main elements of PACE were 16 local projects set up in spring 1996 to explore issues about implementation in relation to a range of clinical topics and a network involving over 500 people working in and with the NHS.

A first report, *Turning Evidence into Everyday Practice*, was published in November 1997 to provide an interim review of progress. This final report builds on that report and provides a more detailed account of the work in the local projects. It suggests action needed to support the continuing development of evidence-based practice in the new NHS. It is based on discussion with those leading the local projects, their final project reports and the findings from an independent evaluation undertaken by Templeton College.

What is in the report?

Chapter 1 provides background information about the programme overall.

Chapter 2 offers advice about the essential tasks involved in implementing change in clinical practice – drawing on examples of the work in the local projects and related research evidence about the effectiveness of these techniques. It also suggests how organisations can draw on the lessons from the programme to develop a practical, integrated approach to clinical governance.

Chapter 3 describes the work undertaken in the 16 local projects and explains why the projects were established, the evidence base for the work, what happened in the projects and what changed and the impact the work has had so far on local clinical practice.

The Appendix provides contact details for the 16 local projects.

Who is this report for?

This report has been designed to help people working in and with the NHS, who are concerned to improve the quality of care for patients. In particular, it should be of help to people in:

Commissioning – in health authorities and primary care groups; for example, as they draw up health improvement plans and local commissioning strategies to secure the best use of resources.

Providing care to patients – in primary and secondary care; for example, as local initiatives are being developed to help clinicians use research evidence as part of their clinical decision-making and to develop local arrangements for clinical governance.

Patient groups and organisations, who are working with local health services to help ensure that local practice is responsive to the needs of patients.

Professional organisations, as they develop support for the concept of lifelong learning, as described in the consultative paper *A First Class Service*.

Professional education, as they teach the health care practitioners of tomorrow.

Research and development, so that they can understand the challenges involved in using research findings to improve services to patients and can develop approaches to the dissemination of the results of their work.

How can the report be used?

By *individuals* – as a source of information about the implementation of evidence-based practice.

In *project work* – as a template against which those who are planning a project approach to implementation can compare their own plans and identify ideas based on the experience in the local projects which may help them take their projects forward.

For team building – as support in the development of multi-disciplinary working by providing examples to help clarify roles and contributions in the implementation of change in clinical practice.

In *organisational development* – to illustrate how integration of local systems (audit, information, education, etc.) can support the delivery of evidence-based practice.

The report is intended to be used either as a basis for *self-assessment*, i.e. to allow people to judge how well they are doing, or as the basis for *peer review*, i.e. by offering a framework within which an external team could be invited to assess the development of local projects and/or organisations. Chapter 2 offers a series of questions that can be addressed in this review process.

Chapter 1

Setting the context

The background to PACE

PACE was set up in 1995 and arose out of growing concern at that time about the lack of understanding about how to implement change in clinical practice. Significant research endeavour had over the years been devoted to questions in this field, but the findings from this research were equivocal. One factor was however clear – a multi-faceted approach using a number of linked activities was most likely to be successful. Meanwhile, some local development projects were starting to show that local success in achieving change in clinical practice was possible.

The linked objectives for the programme were to: support a number of local 'demonstration' projects focused on the implementation of evidence-based practice; support a network of individuals who had an interest in clinical effectiveness; and disseminate the lessons from the local projects.

The aim was to build on the experience of managing implementation activities, the lessons about managing change and the emerging evidence about changing clinical behaviour. The three-year programme was based at the King's Fund and financial support provided by the NHS Executive. Over the three years about £1.2 million was allocated to support the programme. This covered grants to the local projects and the costs for the PACE team at the King's Fund, publications and meetings.

This report builds on the interim report from the programme, *Turning Evidence into Everyday Practice*, which was published in November 1997. It does not, however, repeat all the detailed material in that report, such as lessons about working with primary care and information about the work of the Network.

The programme was completed, as scheduled, by the end of December 1998.

Support for the local projects

The projects covered a variety of clinical topics and a wide range of local organisations, health authorities, NHS trusts, audit groups and primary care. Moreover, the projects were at different stages of development, with some closely linked to local development work. In this report a 'shorthand' reference, for example, to the location of the projects, is used rather than titles that embrace all the organisations involved.

The local teams were supported through two parallel activities:

- *a series of project group meetings* which enabled representatives from the local projects to meet and share their experiences. These meetings included presentations by the projects and small group discussions focused on current issues. For example, in the early stages of the project work one of these meetings was devoted to issues about involving patients in the project work. Over the life of the projects eight project group meetings were organised. Information about the main points from these discussions was used to produce the regular *PACE Bulletin*.

- *regular visits to the local projects*. Concentrated in the early stages of the work, these were opportunities to review progress and identify emerging issues that might merit attention at the project group meetings. The local project teams were encouraged to use the visits and their own meetings as opportunities for reflection to ensure that the learning from the work was captured. The visits also provided opportunities to review ideas about how best to measure the impact of the local projects and about how to disseminate the learning from the local project work. Throughout the programme the emphasis for the PACE team was on providing advice and support rather than playing an active role in the local projects.

Aspects of evaluation

The work undertaken within the programme was evaluated through three parallel activities:

- an *'action learning'* approach was adopted to identify the emerging lessons from the work, for example, in the project group meetings
- a team based at Templeton College, Oxford, was commissioned by the NHS Executive to provide an *independent assessment* of how the changes were achieved by the local projects. The results of that work are reflected in this report and a report of their study will also be published
- arrangements were made to support action by the projects to *measure the impact* of their work. This aspect is described in more detail in the following paragraphs.

Three activities supported the action learning approach:

- the regular visits to, and meetings with, the local project teams
- discussions at project group meetings, particularly in July 1997 and July 1998, i.e. at a mid-point in the projects' timetables and as they were coming to an end

- mid-term and final project reports produced by the project leaders. A common structure was adopted for these reports; for example, the final reports covered the techniques and change mechanisms used, the arrangements for managing the work, notes on factors for success, the approach to self-assessment and reflection adopted during the project and plans for using the learning from the project in other clinical settings.

In addition, the emerging findings from the independent evaluation being undertaken by the Templeton College guided the preparation of the interim and final reports. All the information assembled through these activities was systematically analysed to identify the key themes and lessons and thus enable reports to be prepared.

The aspect of the evaluation focused on measuring concentrated on the process of change rather than the outcome of change: a reflection of the main objective of the programme which was to implement proven interventions rather than to prove, again, their effectiveness. The main objective was thus to monitor the application of the recommended interventions, treatments or procedures. Those projects requiring a more detailed assessment of impact were encouraged to use published outcomes to 'estimate' the expected local effect. For some projects this approach was problematic and concerns were raised about attribution of cause and effect. Some projects employed the services of local academic units, particularly for economic assessment.

The PACE team worked with the project teams to identify a 'basket' of indicators using, where possible, routinely collected data such as PACT and HES. Local project teams were also invited to identify comparison data in order to see whether implementation had achieved anything more than the changes that might have happened anyway. A set of principles were developed to guide these discussions. These included:

- rely on the original research to demonstrate benefit
- focus on the process of implementation rather than on researching outcomes
- rely, wherever possible, on routine data
- establish baseline data against which to measure change
- identify suitable comparison data
- develop a process to monitor the indicators.

In addition, the following questions were identified to help local projects in taking forward their plans for measurement:

- are relevant routine data available?

- can clinical audit provide any information on, say, baseline activity?
- if a more specific assessment of outcome is required, is it possible to estimate the local outcome by applying the results from published research?
- if customised data are required, are they prohibitively difficult and/or expensive to collect and analyse?

Turning Evidence into Everyday Practice identified a number of cautionary notes about the impact measurement aspects of the programme and specifically about:

- *attribution*, and the problems of being sure that any change had occurred because of the project
- the *natural history of diseases* and the time frame for PACE
- data collection and use of *routine information systems*.

The impact of the projects, within the timescale of the programme, is illustrated in Chapter 3, but to ensure that this report was published on time, a line had to be drawn in terms of data collection in the summer of 1998. For some projects this was probably 'too early' because of the nature of their work. While some encouraging changes can be reported, it has become clear that the information currently available represents only the start of the story. A further assessment of the impact of the projects would add significantly to future debates about the effectiveness of action to change clinical practice.

Support to the PACE Network

The Network provided a means through which members could share their experiences, learn about initiatives being taken forward elsewhere and meet colleagues with similar interests. It was launched in January 1996 and ran until July 1998. Over 500 members, including clinicians, managers, clinical audit staff and researchers joined.

The main features of the Network were a database of members' interests, a regular bulletin and a programme of Network Discussion Days. From the outset the aim was to be proactive and provide opportunities for members to meet, rather than relying on the circulation of lists of members and expect individuals to follow up common interests.

Between July 1996 and July 1998, 50 Discussion Days were organised involving about 700 participants – members and their colleagues. The topics for discussion included clinical areas (such as cardiac care and diabetes) as well as generic questions (such as 'how to create a clinical effectiveness strategy'). The sessions enabled members to learn about both the work being taken forward by others and the emerging lessons from the local projects. Notes were circulated to remind those involved of some of the main points from the discussions. Evaluation showed that these sessions were helpful to and popular with members.

Disseminating the learning from the local projects

From the outset, the aim of PACE was to share the lessons from the work as the programme was taken forward, rather than waiting until the programme was completed. This approach was adopted because of the scale of interest in the implementation of evidence-based practice. A variety of ways were adopted to publicise the work.

The programme was launched with the publication of the first issue of the *PACE Bulletin* in September 1995. The bulletin was then published quarterly to report on progress with the programme overall, the key messages from the projects and progress with the Network. The bulletin was designed in a simple two-page, easy-to-read format and included reports which provided short headline messages to encourage contact with the PACE team, membership of the Network and/or contact with the local projects.

In addition, in 1996, a series of discussion papers about aspects of implementation were made available. These were designed to complement the headlines in the bulletin. *Turning Evidence into Everyday Practice* was published in November 1997 to report on progress about half way through the programme. The lessons emerging from the work were also disseminated through articles in journals and presentations at conferences.

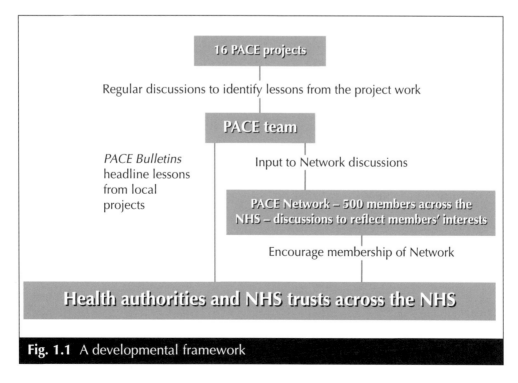

Fig. 1.1 A developmental framework

The approach was deliberately participative: to show that the programme had something to offer others interested in implementing evidence-based practice. The separate components of the programme – the projects, network and dissemination activities – were designed as a developmental framework to add strength to the individual components (see Fig. 1.1). Experience has shown that the framework enhanced the impact of the individual components.

Chapter 2

Building on the evidence, learning from experience

This chapter brings together the practical experience and lessons learned by the local projects with the emerging research evidence about changing clinical practice and organisational development. It draws on the lessons from managing the local projects, using examples and comments from the project reports to the King's Fund and references for useful sources and relevant research. The chapter addresses, first, what needs to be done and follows this with points about managing the work. The final section suggests how managing implementation in the 'new NHS' might be developed.

Further information about the projects is available from the contacts listed in the Appendix.

Experience, evidence and knowledge

The work in the local projects over the last two years, and discussions with those involved in similar work, have identified three essential attributes of successful management of implementation initiatives. These are: awareness of the emerging *evidence* about changing clinical behaviour and organisational development; the value of *experience* of managing change in the Health Service; and the need for local *knowledge* and understanding of organisational structures and relationships. This chapter draws on:

- the experience of and lessons learned by those leading the local projects
- the independent evaluation of PACE by a team based at Templeton College, Oxford
- the work of the Cochrane Effective Practice and Organisation of Care group (EPOC)
- research focused on the development of organisations.

The PACE experience demonstrates that:

- *implementation is a messy business.* The key words are facilitation and flexibility with the project leaders needing to coax, cajole and drive the work forward. *'Be prepared to encounter resistance from unexpected quarters'* – Oxfordshire. *'Progress of the project was more evolutionary and incremental than deadline-focused'* – Barnet.

- *implementation is not a linear task.* There are no distinctly separate stages to the work, but rather it depends upon a group of inter-related tasks that require skill, dexterity and resources to manage to a satisfactory conclusion. The experience has reaffirmed the message from research that a multi-faceted approach, using a range of techniques, can be successful.

- *implementation takes time.* No matter how well a plan is prepared, the work is likely to take longer than expected! It takes time to assemble evidence, to arrange meetings involving busy clinicians, to prepare material for and to arrange training courses – again for busy clinicians – and to set up discussions with patients and carers, etc. *North Derbyshire suggested that the sensible thing to do was create a plan and then double the time allowed. 'We wouldn't expect to devise a credible implementation programme for evidence-based change in primary care in under a year'* – Bromley.

- *implementation is expensive.* It requires a significant commitment if success is to be achieved. All the projects received a grant of £30,000 over two years to support the work, but this represented only a small part of the 'cost'. *Experience from Dudley suggests that delivering their project had involved about 500 working days – of which only about a fifth was 'paid for' by the project grant.*

The experience has, however, shown that this effort is worthwhile. Improvements to the care and treatment of patients have been achieved. *'It was sobering to meet people suffering from a painful and debilitating condition, who had received largely ineffective care for almost as long as the NHS had existed. The continuing resolve of everyone concerned is to ensure that people receive the care and services they need to improve the quality of their lives'* – Royal Berkshire.

Moreover, the projects have enabled many people to develop new skills and working relationships and the 'costs' involved should be seen as an investment. *'After the steep learning curve the task gets easier'* – Dorset. Many of the projects have been the catalyst for a range of related activities, such as the development of local implementation programmes covering a range of clinical conditions. *'PACE education' is a name now used in Bradford to describe a series of events for primary care groups.*

Ten essential tasks

Ten essential, and often overlapping, tasks require attention if success in implementing change is to be achieved. These tasks need to be viewed as separate components of one bigger task, rather than a series of discrete, independent activities. Figure 2.1 illustrates the overall aim of implementing change as a wall with each task pictured as a brick. For example, while attention to the choice of topic and engaging clinicians will create a sound foundation for future work, action at an early stage to explore questions about how to secure change and how to measure it would be sensible. The main challenge is to keep the overall activity in mind and not concentrate too narrowly on the separate tasks. Avoid the notion of steps, but bear in mind that some of the tasks will be ongoing and require attention throughout the initiative, while other tasks will be time-limited.

Each of the tasks is examined in the following paragraphs and, for each, a set of questions is suggested to facilitate the review of local implementation activities.

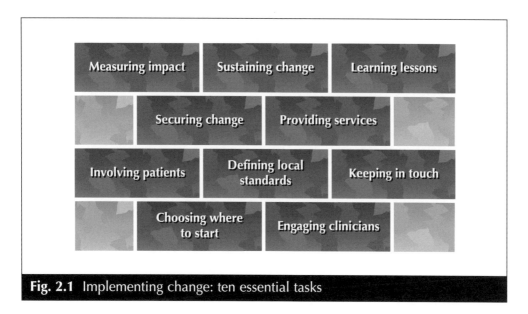

Fig. 2.1 Implementing change: ten essential tasks

Choosing where to start should be treated seriously because of the challenging nature of implementation. Before preliminary local investigations are set in hand, arrangements need to be agreed and put in place for *how* the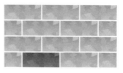
decision will be made, i.e. *who* will be involved, at *what* level in the organisation and *who* will handle discussions with partner organisations (the health authority, local primary care groups, local trusts, etc.). Preparatory work can be managed in five stages.

1. Establishing criteria to facilitate the choice of topic. Two main factors to consider are:

- concern expressed by clinicians about the quality of current practice, awareness of unmet need and the need for change. This might have been demonstrated in a recent clinical audit study. *North Derbyshire was able to build on strong concern expressed by local GPs about the quality of care being provided to patients with congestive cardiac failure*
- recognition by senior management that change is required, with consequent support for the initiative, and the possible need for additional resources.

In addition, until local experience in successfully concluding implementation initiatives has been acquired, it would be helpful to consider:

- the conclusions from earlier work – what progress was made and why was that work not maintained? *South Tyneside was able to build on successful related initiatives which had built excellent working relationships particularly between MAAG and practices*
- strong local working relationships and knowledge of the 'patch', which would facilitate the work – and good teamwork
- involvement of a wide range of disciplines. This would secure broad impact – for example, to ensure that a range of disciplines in a number of organisations are involved.

2. Assembling the evidence to underpin the work. A set of evidence-based guidelines or the evidence presented following a systematic review should be a starting point, rather than seeking locally to assemble primary research evidence. '*The presence of "rock solid evidence" greatly improves the chance of persuading doctors and other health professional to change'* – Templeton evaluation report. '*It is unlikely that a local group would have been able to produce a scientifically based document'* – Barnet.

Over the last few years the UK Cochrane Centre, the NHS Centre for Reviews and Dissemination and other similar bodies have started to improve access to evidence. The planned work programme for the proposed National Institute of Clinical Excellence should add to this. The use of critical appraisal training can help to develop people's understanding of the nature of research evidence.

3. Assessing current practice. The potential scale and nature of change need to be established, specifically to identify clinical staff whose practice may need to change. At this stage a broad illustration of the scale of change is required, not necessarily a detailed picture of local practice. A preliminary audit, based on draft practice standards, may be helpful. *A district-wide audit in North Derbyshire demonstrated that, although results reported were better than results reported elsewhere, they did not reach acceptable standards and helped to secure support for the need to improve the care and treatment of patients with congestive cardiac failure.*

4. Determining local priorities. Tasks 2 and 3 above will enable the local 'practice gap' (i.e. the difference between current practice and evidence) to be assessed and provide a basis for a local implementation plan.

5. Securing local commitment for the work. Experience in many of the projects has shown that those initiatives that attract and sustain commitment from senior staff in the organisation/s are the more likely to succeed. For example, a willingness to release clinical staff from their duties to attend training sessions and a readiness to redeploy resources to reflect changed demands on services.

Key sources: Evidence and guidelines

– *Cochrane Library.* Website: http://hiru.mcmaster.ca/COCHRANE/DEFAULT.htm
– *NHS Centre for Reviews and Dissemination* (CRD)
  Website: http://www.york.ac.uk/inst/crd/centre.htm
– *Agency for Health Care Policy and Research* – full text versions of guidelines, quick reference guides and patient versions of guidelines can be downloaded from (http://text.nlm.nih.gov/ftrs/dbaccess/ahcpr) or ordered from the AHCPR website (http://www.ahcpr.gov/cgi-bin/gilssrch.pl). (AHCPR are about to produce a guidelines clearing house on the web – see http://www.ahcpr.gov/clinic/ngcfact.htm for details).
– *Canadian Medical Association Clinical Practice Infobase* – index of clinical practice guidelines; includes downloadable full text versions or abstracts for most guidelines (http://www.cma.ca/cpgs/index.html)
– *Scottish Intercollegiate Guidelines Network* (SIGN) (http://pc47.cee.hw.ac.uk/sign/home.htm)
– *Netting the Evidence.* The ScHARR (Sheffield) Website: http://www.shef.ac.uk/uni/academic/R-K/scharr/ir/netting.html
– *National Guidelines Directory* published by the Royal College of Nursing. RCN Website: http://www.rcn.org.uk
– *Critical Appraisal Skills Programme:* CASP, Institute of Health Sciences, Old Road, Headington Oxford, OX3 7LF. Website: http://www.ihs.ox.ac.uk/casp/noframes/casp.html

Question to address: Choosing where to start

* Will action in the chosen topic attract commitment and command local support?
  – particularly from *clinicians* likely to be affected; and
  – from *senior managers* who may need to meet the resource consequences of the work.
* Have any audits been undertaken that can tell you about current practice?
* What is the scale and nature of change required?

* What are the expected health benefits of change?
* Is a reputable review of relevant research and/or national evidence-based guidelines available?
* Are critical appraisal skills locally available?

Engaging clinicians and establishing strong and lasting working relationships provide a valuable basis for future activity. Clinicians' support for the work is essential. Action on four aspects needs to be considered.

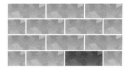

1. Understanding the local context. Established approaches to managing change emphasise the need for contextual analysis, i.e. a sustained effort to understand local processes, relationships and likely resistance to change. A variety of approaches were adopted in the local projects to help them identify local organisational and professional factors and understand the needs of individuals. *However, the Templeton evaluation reported that several projects doubted the wisdom of formalising their assessment of the individuals concerned – for example, by creating a detailed analysis and thus labelling people (as either likely to be supportive – or likely to be difficult!). Experience has shown that reliance on a broad assessment, rather than a detailed one, has been adequate.*

2. Identifying local clinical leaders. The experiences in the projects have shown that the engagement of senior local clinicians, to provide clinical leadership, was an important factor for success. Several projects identified individual clinicians and managers who proved to be valuable leaders, allies and project 'champions'. Some of these emerged as the work was taken forward, rather than before the work started. Therefore, do not label people unless you are sure about their response to the work: expect the unexpected. Local clinical leaders are not necessarily the same as 'opinion leaders', i.e. those who are nominated by their peers and who are educationally influential. The latter have been the subject of extensive research but the findings are inconclusive.

A leadership role within the project will place a significant burden on clinicians and ways may need to be found to provide support to free up their time. Throughout, it is important to develop good working relationships. *'Personal relationships were vital, with trust and honesty prerequisites to progress at practice level'* – LSL/King's.

3. Recognising potential barriers to change. A number of research studies have offered possible approaches to categorising barriers to change. For example, one approach suggests four categories which may require attention:

* *cultural,* when conflicting local or organisational priorities may hinder efforts to secure support of senior management. Moreover, there may be little experience or

history in multi-disciplinary team working. Characteristically, clinical effectiveness activities span several clinical and managerial disciplines.

- *organisational*, delivery of effective care requires an organisation-wide approach built on integration of local systems. Prevailing fragmentation among groups (e.g. doctors, nurses, and managers) and local systems (e.g. audit, education, training and library systems) is also an obstacle to change.

- *personal*, clinical staff may be sceptical about the merit of evidence-based practice, particularly if they have practised for many years without problems: they may ask 'what does evidence offer me?'. The work may also require unfamiliar skills such as critical appraisal of research literature, communication methods and measuring outcomes. This scepticism may extend also to doubts about the 'evidence' being implemented. Criticisms may include the fact that the evidence has limited applicability, especially where the evidence has an impact across different clinical divides. There may also be a perception of loss of clinical freedom.

- *resource-related*, implementation is a resource-intensive activity. It requires time, resources and, almost certainly, change to local services. Many clinicians may feel that they simply do not have the time or money to become involved.

Identifying and reviewing how these barriers can be overcome will be an important step in developing an implementation plan.

4. *Presenting information carefully*. Avoid creating the impression that the initiative is a threat to clinicians. Bear in mind that they will believe that they are doing the best that they can and information about the initiative should be presented, as part of their continuing professional development, and thus in ways that promote professionalism. The Government's proposals for 'lifelong learning' set out in A *First Class Service* may provide a future context for 'engaging clinicians'.

Key references: Engaging clinicians _____

- *Managing change*. Garside P. Organisational context for quality: lessons from the fields of organisational development and change management. Quality in Health Care 1998; 7 (Suppl):S1–S2
- *Opinion Leaders*. Thompson *et al*. 1997. Cochrane Library.
  Website: http://hiru.mcmaster.ca/COCHRANE/DEFAULT.htm
- *Barriers*. Lomas J. Teaching old (and not so old) doctors new tricks: effective ways to implement research findings. In: Dunn EV, Norton PG, Stewart M, Tudiver F, Bass MJ (eds). Disseminating research/changing practice. Research methods for Primary Care. Volume 6. Sage Publications, Thousand Oaks, 1994

*Questions to address: Engaging clinicians*_____

* Have you identified those clinicians and managers who will be affected – directly or indirectly – by the proposal?
* Have you considered how those affected will react to the proposal?
* Are the most influential clinicians involved in developing the proposal?
* Have the likely barriers to change, along with realistic ways to overcome them, been identified?

Involving patients is an imperative in these 'consumerist' times. There is a patchy body of evidence in this field, but the evidence available suggests that involving patients in decisions about their care and treatment can lead to better outcomes. As work is taken forward, three aspects merit attention.

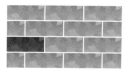

*1. Being clear about **why** patients are involved in the project.* The projects have sought involvement at two levels: at an individual level in patients' own care and treatment and/or at a collective strategic level to influence service planning and delivery. Reasons for involvement can range from wanting to provide information about effective treatments and raising awareness about services, to using patients' views to improve services. *In Dudley, focus groups showed that women prefer to discuss incontinence with a woman, and a nurse rather than a doctor. On a broader level, local initiatives sought to raise awareness of the condition and the fact that there was effective treatment available. 'Many of the problems arose here from the embarrassing and stigmatising nature of the condition.'*

Face-to-face meetings between patients and clinicians were an effective mechanism for changing clinical behaviour. *LSL/King's used a series of focus groups to explore what was effective from a patient's perspective. They subsequently found that patients could be useful change agents. Changes introduced covered aspects of care (such as involving families and carers) and aspects of consultations (such as explaining the purpose of investigations). 'It is possible to work with patients and gain valuable insights into their values and concepts of clinical effectiveness. Their views may challenge the scientific approach to effectiveness. The process is not expensive and is fairly straightforward.'*

*2. Determining **how** to involve patients.* This means being clear about whom to involve and creating the right mechanisms to do so. The community health council, voluntary sector or patient and carer groups may provide useful sources of expertise and help in accessing the views of users. Bear in mind that the views of some groups (e.g. patients, carers, the public) may not always be consistent. Identifying appropriate mechanisms for gathering information – whether through focus groups, local surveys or other means – is another step towards assembling information about patients' views on current services. *In South Tyneside, a patient-held record was produced following patient and clinician focus group discussions. 'We felt this would be a major change mechanism and a principal focus of patient involvement, though defining the role of patients has been problematic. The feedback from patient focus groups was illuminating and helped to reinforce aims and objectives of the project'.* Many of the later points about 'keeping in touch' (see pp. 17–19) are also important when 'involving patients'.

*3. Ensuring that patients **are** involved.* A lay representative on the project team can ensure that patient involvement is not an afterthought. *In Wirral a service user was involved in the project steering group and a carers' group provided advice.* When developing patient information, patients need to be involved in the process of production and thought needs to be given to integrating systems in order to get the materials to patients. *Bromley aimed to get patients to contribute to creating information leaflets about H. pylori eradication but it was difficult to recruit a suitable group of patients. Instead, they identified material developed elsewhere and adapted it in discussion with local clinicians. The patient information now sits alongside related material in the patients' medical record and is designed to be given to patients as prescribing decisions are made. In Dudley, patients were invited to help with translations and innovative ways tried to reach people, for example, 'toilet stickers' in the public toilets in health care premises to provide contact details for the continence service: 'One needs to keep the message simple, get the language and presentation right and be sensitive to community languages translation problems and cultural differences'.*

Key sources: Involving patients

- *Informing patients: An assessment of the quality of patient information materials.* Coulter A, Entwistle V, Gilbert D. London. King's Fund, 1998.
- *Information for patients:* Centre for Health Information Quality. Winchester SO22 5DH Website: http://www.centreforhiq.demon.co.uk/
- *But will it work doctor? Promoting and supporting patient choice by making evidence about the effectiveness of health care accessible to health service users.* Report of 2nd 'But will it work, doctor?' conference, Northampton. Dunning M, Needham G, Weston S (ed.) 1997. ISBN 1 898300 119.
- *In the public interest: developing a strategy for public participation in the NHS.* NHS Executive, NHS Confederation, Institute for Health Service Management, 1998.

Questions to address: Involving patients

* Are there existing patient information leaflets etc. (produced locally or elsewhere) available which could be used to support your initiative?
* How are you going to ensure that you involve people from all parts of the local community and the 'hard to reach'? (e.g. minority ethnic groups)
* Have previous activities (on patient involvement) been reviewed to provide a basis for discussions on planned new initiatives – what went well and what didn't?

* Which local self-help groups, patient organisations and/or voluntary organisations' representatives could contribute to the work?

Defining local standards will help create a sound base for the initiative by providing clarity about the intended quality of practice. Three aspects merit attention.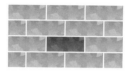

1. Deciding how standards will be presented. Local sensitivities should dictate whether these are presented as 'guidelines', 'pathways' or 'clinical management protocols'. *North Derbyshire decided to present information to GPs in a practice information pack rather than as a set of guidelines because they were keen to focus on the evidence base for the work, rather than the presentation of a guideline. Gloucestershire Royal chose to develop a care pathway because it would support their longer-term aim to introduce an electronic patient record. Walsall chose to present their proposed standard as a clinical management pathway because of local antagonism to guidelines.*

2. Creating guidelines. Extensive research has demonstrated that properly developed and disseminated clinical guidelines can encourage clinicians to change their practice. Guidelines are more likely to be effective if they take into account local circumstances and are complemented by suitable educational activities and active implementation strategies, such as the creation of patient-specific reminders.

Most of the projects included the creation of local guidelines, with many built on published national guidelines. The task of tailoring guidelines for local use can be time-consuming and it is important to balance the effort devoted to this task. *'In the absence of national guidelines the amount of time and expertise required to put together local guidelines should not be underestimated'* – Chase Farm. Because of the skills and resources required to create evidence-based guidelines, it is wise to build on such work already undertaken elsewhere.

Aim to create a guideline that is 'good enough' rather than 'the best'. Experience has shown that guidelines should be visually attractive, but not over-elaborate. *'Clear messages in the guidelines, with the evidence displayed and graded, was seen as very influential'* – Bradford. Remember to put in place arrangements to keep guidelines up to date: they soon become out of date as current research is completed, reviewed and published.

3. Demonstrating the benefits of change. The analysis of current practice set alongside draft local standards should inform statements about the scale of change proposed and the benefits of the work for clinical staff (the impact on their clinical time, etc.) and for patients. Both of these can be helpful as work is taken forward to overcome barriers and resistance to change. *Bromley 'placed evidence of divergent current practice alongside specific research evidence' as a means of securing support for the development of guidelines and the need for change.*

Key references and sources: Defining local standards _____

- *Implementing clinical guidelines.* Effective Health Care. Bulletin No 8. Leeds, University of Leeds, 1994.
- *Assessing Guidelines.* Service funded by NHS Executive to quality-assured nationally developed guidelines. Website: http://www.sghms.ac.uk/depts/phs/hceu/nhsguide.htm

Questions to address: Defining local standards _____

* Have you reviewed, with local clinicians, how standards should be presented?
* Have relevant existing local and national guidelines been identified?
* What problems have been encountered in promoting earlier local guidelines?
* Are local guidelines consistent (i.e. with no conflict between the 'new' and established ones)?
* Do the plans to develop guidelines accord with proven good practice?
* Are mechanisms available to keep standards up to date after they have been developed? How will such changes be disseminated?

Keeping in touch with local staff – clinicians and managers – who will be affected by the initiative will help to smooth the path for the work.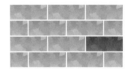

1. Taking communications seriously. The work is likely to have an impact across clinical and managerial staff so action to keep everyone informed about the work is important. Positive steps can ensure that staff understand the impact of the work, how the work affects them and how it is progressing. Other action (on engaging clinicians) will have established an understanding of who will be *involved* and those who will need to be kept *informed,* i.e. those whose interests are indirect, such as senior managers.

Most of the projects had strategies to guide their communication efforts. '*A strategy was agreed to inform colleagues of work in progress and to consult them as the care pathway was being developed*' – *Gloucestershire Royal.* Several projects that had not formulated a communications strategy recognised that it would have facilitated progress if they had done so as an early part of their work.

2. Being clear about the messages and the role of the messenger. Experience has shown the advantages of focusing on clear, simple and consistent messages, which evolve as work on the project progresses, and judging with care who will be entrusted with carrying the message. *'As the project progressed, it became clear that a single consistent message to GPs was vital. Different messages from different gynaecological teams was undermining the credibility of the local guidelines'* – Dorset. *'Project team members took individual responsibility for monitoring the effectiveness of communications with their own [disciplinary] group'* – Royal Berkshire. *'Be prepared to repeat and reinforce the information: absence of that reinforcement – even for a short time – can lead to rapid back-sliding'* – Oxfordshire.

It has proven helpful in some projects to have one individual as a point of contact for the project – although if that person is not full time, contingency arrangements need to be made for when that person is not available. *'Difficulties could have arisen if the secretarial staff had not been conscientious in their receiving and passing on of messages'* – North Derbyshire.

3. *Using existing communication systems.* This will save time and avoid adding to existing meeting schedules and documentation. *'Existing channels were used: team briefings, practice nurse meetings, GP newsletters and the trust professional forum'* – Wigan and Bolton. *'The sheer size of the problem threatened to overwhelm us. There were literally thousands of people who we felt needed to know about the project. The cost of producing a project newsletter would have been prohibitive – and there was still the problem of trying to get people to read it!'* – Royal Berkshire.

4. *Enlisting the support of allies.* Allies should include those in contact with clinicians whose practice may need to change; for example, prescribing advisers can reinforce messages in their discussions with GPs. Similarly, it is helpful to consider the role of others in direct contact with patients, such as community pharmacists and GP tutors. It is essential to ensure that allies carry consistent messages about the project and the standards of practice being sought.

North Derbyshire broke new ground locally in involving community pharmacists in this type of work. Other local development work has since benefited from their involvement and community pharmacists have been able to contribute to debates about the establishment of primary care groups. In Wigan and Bolton, the role that community pharmacists could play in supporting the continence service was examined. A training session was subsequently organised to ensure that community pharmacists understood the aims of the project and were able to give their customers appropriate advice on the promotion of continence.

Questions to address: Keeping in touch

* Are you clear about *what* you need to communicate and *to whom* the message is relevant?
* Have you prepared a simple and concise note to ensure messages are consistent (and established ways of keeping this up to date as the project progresses)?

* Have you reviewed existing communications channels to identify the best ways of reaching those affected by the project?
* Have you assigned responsibility for communications to appropriate members of the project team – to keep in touch with their peers?
* Have you identified allies, other colleagues regularly in touch with those who will be affected, and who could help reinforce your messages?
* Have you established mechanisms for monitoring the effectiveness of your communications?

Securing change will require attention to six inter-linked activities. This task will consume the largest share of resources (time and people) available for the work.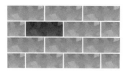

1. Being incremental. An understanding of the local context will provide valuable intelligence on which to base the project work. However, experience has shown the benefit of tackling the work incrementally, starting with a local 'pilot group' of clinicians to test out the proposed approach. *A group of six general practices were chosen at random to test the approach being developed in Bromley. 'Piloting change was a valuable process. It was a chance to ensure that the process for driving change works ... We could talk credibly about its flexibility and applicability in a range of different practices' – Bromley. 'The incremental build-up of the different aspects of the project has allowed time for each activity to be developed and understood before the next one was introduced' – North Derbyshire.* The project timetable should allow time to review the experience in the separate stages of the work *before* the project is rolled forward.

2. Enlisting the support of clinical leaders. There is an important role for respected clinical leaders to help spread the message about the work and what is involved. *The Templeton evaluation report suggests that there can be a mutually reinforcing relationship between evidence and local experts: the endorsement of evidence by a local clinical leader can make the evidence more credible. Experience has shown that the absence of a local clinical leader can be a major obstacle.* But it has proven to be important to realise also that 'new' leaders can be identified as the project work evolves rather than believe that they can be identified at the outset. *'It proved helpful to enrol staff from pilot sites as champions as the project was rolled out' – Dudley.*

3. Supporting the development of multi-disciplinary teams. Research has demonstrated that teams can produce better patient care. Effective teams have shown that they provide a means to harness the different contributions of individual clinical disciplines to the best effect for patients. The development of such teams requires the shared ownership of a common purpose, clarity about the contributions made by each discipline and an essential need for open communications between team members. Teams also provide a way through which individuals can enhance their own clinical skills.

In the projects a common understanding of the relevant research and evidence was an important factor. *Gloucestershire Royal had to secure cross-disciplinary agreement about the nature and basis of respective contributions to patient care to enable the development of the integrated care pathway to go ahead. In Wirral the project team chose to manage the integration of the family support worker (who was employed through a local voluntary organisation – Making Space) into the community psychiatric nurses team in ways which would identify lessons for the development of other teams. Important points emerging from the discussions in Wirral included:*

- *ensuring that each member of the team retained a **separate function** and thus avoided the need to examine the different skills and common abilities of team members*
- *ensuring **joint training** on the aims for the new service; this was difficult because different agencies (both statutory – health and social services – and voluntary organisations) were responsible for different staff within the team*
- *ensuring that **inter-disciplinary tensions** were seen as a positive contribution to patient care: staff were encouraged to advocate on the care of clients from their own professional base and thus increase the debate about options for care.*

More generally, a number of projects saw a team approach as a means of encouraging more cautious members to consider and adopt an evidence-based approach to their contribution to patient care.

4. Providing education and training opportunities. Clinical staff need to be allowed to reflect on current local practice and how the use of research evidence could improve quality. *'The main tool adopted for the management of the change process has been education and training'* – Wirral. Research suggests that interactive training sessions are more likely to change clinical practice than lectures but some of the projects have included presentations by local consultants as part of an overall programme. They were seen as an important way of demonstrating their role in and support for the work. Such sessions offered an important means of developing links and personal contacts between primary and secondary care. *'We consider the formal presentation by a consultant to be emblematic to GPs – until more effective ways of postgraduate education and training become the norm'* – Walsall.

As plans for training sessions are being developed, training needs should be assessed and ways developed to meet those needs. Be clear who needs to be involved. *'Educational programmes need to be imaginative, flexible and tailored to the needs of staff'* – Chase Farm. Three levels of training need were identified in Royal Berkshire: the need for **specialist** knowledge to assess and draw up a protocol for individual patient treatment, for **practitioner** level to handle day-to-day treatment within the protocol and **general awareness** of the resource and treatment issues relating to leg ulcers. Barnet found that by offering

educational support to general practices they were able to raise the profile from a marketing exercise to an educational, and thus change, initiative.

Training programmes should respond to the needs of the individuals and the organisation and ensure that clinical staff can be released from clinical duties. Experience has shown that practice-based training sessions and providing one-to-one, face-to-face tuition have been effective, although time-consuming. *'It was impossible to provide formal teaching sessions to groups of nurses because they could not be released from clinical duties: tuition was provided on a one-to-one basis' – Oxfordshire. 'The main thrust of the outreach nurse's job was to explain the project and catalyse the work by the existing team, not to do the work' – LSL/King's.* Appropriate professional accreditation should be obtained for the local sessions. *Dorset enabled GPs to claim CPME points for practice-based training sessions.*

A spin-off from the educational sessions organised as part of the South Tyneside project was the identification of barriers and opportunities which could be taken into account as the project was rolled forward. Similarly, 'regular evaluation of the education sessions ensured that the focus and relevance of the work was maintained' – Chase Farm.

'The most successful educational strategies were those targeted at individual and practice level, which sought to root changes in the reality of GPs' experience and fit in with their way of working' – Templeton evaluation report.

5. *Developing audit tools.* Since the introduction of clinical audit there has been a growing body of experience in the development and management of audit methodologies. The National Centre for Clinical Audit provides a national information service and a mechanism for the sharing of good audit practice. Research has demonstrated that the feedback of the findings from audit studies was most likely to influence clinical practice if it was part of a strategy to target decision-makers who had already agreed to review their practice.

Many of the local projects used audit methodologies as part of their work and experience has shown it made an important contribution, for example, in demonstrating the need for and the benefits of change and in monitoring progress.

In South Tyneside, presentation of audit results to practices was effective in highlighting current shortcomings in practice. In Chase Farm, a documentation audit was undertaken as part of their work to improve record-keeping. Royal Berkshire used an audit of the care and treatment of a group of patients to demonstrate that graduated compression was clinically effective for leg ulcers. The results of the audit were used to promote the benefits of the project locally. Southern Derbyshire introduced arrangements for auditing new patients seen by physiotherapists to monitor to application of the local guidelines. In North Derbyshire, a high level of participation was achieved – for audits by practices – because practices were offered either payment for doing the audit themselves or the services of an audit nurse.

Many of the projects used audit methodologies to review the impact of their work. Some of the results of these audits are reported in Chapter 3.

6. *Providing support to help change happen.* Recognise that implementing change is likely – at least in the early stages – to involve extra work for clinical staff whose time may already be stretched. '*Practice nurses were reluctant to express an interest in the project until they were clear what extra work it would mean for them … Something has to give – health professionals feel that they do not have free time for something new – no matter how important*' – *Dudley.*

Find ways to offer help – for example, to identify existing patients whose treatment may require review and to be clear who will undertake the discussion with patients. '*Many practices were under-using their computer systems. Practice visits helped to identify cardiac populations and create computerised mechanisms for audit and review*' – *LSL/King's.* Pharmaceutical companies may be eager to be involved and offer funding but agree in advance the basis for their contribution. '*Various companies were invited to provide refreshments at training sessions – in return for the opportunity to promote their products. It was stipulated that the product should not be related to the project work*' – *Dorset.*

Key references and sources: Securing change

– *Educational methods.* Davis AD *et al.* Changing physician performance: a systematic review of the effect of continuing medical education strategies. JAMA 1995; 274:700–5.
– *Outreach visits.* Thompson *et al.* 1997. Cochrane Library.
  Website: http://hiru.mcmaster.ca/COCHRANE/DEFAULT.htm
– *Audit and feedback.* Mugford M *et al.* Effects of feedback of information on clinical practice: a review. BMJ 1991; 303:398–402
– *National Centre for Clinical Audit.* Website: http://www.ncca.org.uk/shared/default.htm
– *Team working:*
  – Inter-professional working and continuing medical education. Headrick *et al.* BMJ 7 March 1998; 316:771–4
  – Celebrating teamwork. Firth-Couzens J Quality in Health Care 1998; 7(Suppl):S3–S7

Questions to address: Securing change

* Are the benefits of the proposal for staff *and* patients clear?
* Who needs to change – and how do you plan to approach them? For example, it might be better to approach practice nurses directly rather than via GPs.

* Who can provide clinical leadership for the initiative?
* Have you assessed training needs and reviewed how to develop current local education and training programmes to support the initiative?
* Are people available with the skills to support the delivery of the training programme?
* Have you considered options for supporting the change process, for example to identify patients whose current treatment may require review?
* Have you reviewed – with service managers – arrangements to enable staff to attend briefing and training sessions?
* Have you considered the different ways that clinical audit could support the initiative, for example to illustrate the need for change or to monitor progress?
* Are there audit tools developed and tested elsewhere which could be adopted locally?
* Have you a formal agreement for any involvement by pharmaceutical companies?

Providing services to match planned changes to clinical practice will require a series of parallel actions and experience has shown that this task has been a significant challenge. Points to consider include the following.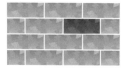

1. Assessing the service and resource consequences of the work. This entails exploring the scale and nature of changes that might be required to reflect the planned changes in practice. An overall lesson was the need to ensure that service managers are included in local discussions from the outset, not only when service consequences are becoming an issue. *In Bromley, the pilot stage of their plan provided valuable local information about the scale of resources needed to implement change on a wider scale. This information was helpful to make a case for additional resources – but even with this information it took many months to secure changes to services.* It is important to assess at the outset what the implications are likely to be. *'The need for pressure care equipment had major cost implications but this was not part of the original project plan' – Chase Farm.*

2. Linking the project to planning and budgeting timetables. Necessary changes to service levels need to go forward hand in hand with changes to practice. The timetable needs to link with local planning and budgeting timetables, but unrealistic expectations should not made about the ability to change practice through the contracting process. *'The project was planned so that services would be in place prior to any increase in demand. A service specification was agreed with the NHS trust' – Wigan and Bolton.*

Experience has shown that the commissioning and contracting system has not necessarily facilitated implementation. *'A clause was inserted in the contract with the NHS trust [about physiotherapy times and priorities] but to date there is no evidence that this clause has impacted on practice' – Southern Derbyshire. In North Derbyshire it proved to be a challenge to work with all the NHS trusts providing services to local residents to assure the development of open-access echocardiography. This involved some trusts where the health authority was not the 'host commissioner' and support from clinicians and managers within the trusts acted as the main catalyst for change.*

Questions to address: Providing services

* Have you reviewed the information available about current services to inform a judgement about the scale and nature of change required?
* Have the costs of any extension to current services been established?
* Are the key service managers involved in the assessment of changes to services?
* Are plans in place to deal with any knock-on budgetary consequences of change?
* Is it possible to set up processes to re-invest savings?

Measuring impact will provide added incentives for the project team as they start to get a feeling of success. Being able to demonstrate achievement is important both for the morale of those involved and to justify service developments. Attention needs to be devoted to two distinct activities.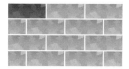

1. Being clear what you need to measure. The effectiveness of the implementation needs checking, rather than to assess the impact on health outcomes. The principles developed to guide the work on measurement within the PACE programme (see Chapter 1) were designed to ensure this focus, i.e. they relied on the original research to show that health outcomes would improve, built on the idea of measuring the process of implementation, and sought to rely as much as possible on routine information systems. An important step in establishing the basis for measuring the impact of the initiative will be to assess with care those aspects of practice that are expected to change.

2. Identifying a suitable 'basket' of measures. A composite picture should be assembled which is capable of monitoring changes across the different aspects of the change process. It is helpful to bring together four or five separate measures which, when taken together, can provide a reliable illustration of the scale and direction of change. This approach will be essential because it is unlikely that implementation will be measurable by one or two direct measures: many NHS information systems do not capture clinical information.

Experience suggests that it is helpful to rely on data to cover prescribing (PACT) as well as hospital activity (HES). It may also be necessary to complement these sources with specific targeted audits. Questions are likely to remain about the extent to which any changes can be attributed to the implementation effort. However, the 'basket' approach should be able to provide confidence about the impact of the work. The impact of the individual local projects is described in Chapter 3.

Questions to address: Measuring impact

* Have you identified the main changes that should flow from the project, such as prescribing levels? Have you reviewed how the information might be collected?
* Is information available from earlier audits that could help identify possible measures?
* Have you identified which routine information systems could support the work?
* Have you reviewed difficulties envisaged in data collection?
* Could other audits provide examples of approaches that might be taken to supplement routine data?

Sustaining change after the project focus has ended will be important to ensure that improvements in practice continue. Action to help to ensure changes endure could include the following.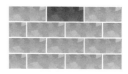

1. Integrating the change into routine care. From the beginning the projects were determined to ensure that the practice improvements which they might achieve would be sustained. Mechanisms were needed to ensure that clinical staff saw the changes as part of the normal routine rather than something special. *'The patient visits [which were introduced by the project] have been devolved to health visitors and district nurses ... integrates these new initiatives into routine care' – LSL/King's.*

2. Ensuring the supply of new documentation. Virtually, all implementation activities will create some new documentation – guidelines, referral forms, protocols, leaflets for patients, etc. Arrangements need to be in place to ensure that supplies are maintained and that clinical staff know where such supplies are held and how they can be obtained.

3. Building reminder systems into patient records. Research has demonstrated the merit of ensuring that reminders of appropriate action are available to clinicians when clinical decisions are made. *'We introduced sticky labels to put on drug charts so it was no trouble to write up a new drug regime' – Oxfordshire.*

4. Providing induction training. High staff turnover suggests that staff induction programmes should be used to ensure that the local practice standards are explained to newly appointed staff. *'When staff leave they take their knowledge with them. In the absence of well-documented and well-implemented systems of care, the main means of sustaining change are repeated education and motivation' – Oxfordshire.*

5. Promoting the achievements. Highlighting success and explaining how the learning is being used in other clinical areas will ensure that interest in the work does not wane. *'PACE education' is a name now used in Bradford to describe a series of events for primary care groups and which will maintain the link between the project and new local initiatives.* The use of regular networks and contacts, such as visits to practices by prescribing advisers can also maintain local interest in the work. *'Working relationships have been built with members of staff from a variety of disciplines and these will help sustain the service developments after the life of the project'* – Dudley. *'The best way of sustaining change is to recognise that your main investment is the people involved'* – Bromley.

Key references: Sustaining change

Reminder systems
- Buntinx F *et al.* Fam Pract 1993; 10:219–28
- Hunt DL, Haynes RB, Hanna SE, Smith K. Effects of computer-based clinical decision support systems on physicians performance and patient outcomes. A systematic review. JAMA 1998; 280, 1339–46.

Questions to address: Sustaining change

* Are arrangements in place to ensure that the induction of new staff reflects the project's objectives?
* Can you ensure the continued supply – after the project work ends – of any material or documents developed as part of the project?
* Are there elements of the changes that could be reinforced by reminder systems as part of patient records?
* Have the changes introduced by the project work been built into existing service and practice monitoring systems?

Learning lessons will help to ensure that other similar, subsequent activities are able to build on the successes *and* failures of the work. It may be helpful to tackle this in two ways.

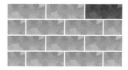

1. Managing the work as a learning process. Arrangements need to be set up to ensure that the lessons learned by individuals and the (project) team are recorded and discussed. Honesty is important. The involvement of someone in the project team with facilitation skills can ensure that time set aside for reflection is used to the optimum effect. Positive action to build an effective team should create a willingness to join in open discussions and, for example, review where things have 'gone wrong' as well as gone well. Do we all learn from mistakes?

A record of key decisions and incidents as the project progresses – a project diary – may be a useful means of maintaining a record of 'successes and failures'. *'As confidence grows, it is important to treat seriously any discomfort or unease with the next stage. Putting off a meeting with a key clinician or not finishing the paperwork for an aspect of the audit may be signs of more serious problems' – Bromley. 'Hidden talents emerged as problems were identified and the team sought to tackle them' – Chase Farm. 'It was clear that practices differed from one another and ways of approaching practices were learned swiftly' – LSL/King's.*

2. *Using the learning.* Experience suggests that the general lessons from the projects are applicable to any work aimed at implementing evidence-based practice – and become increasingly helpful as health care organisations make plans to implement a systematic approach to clinical governance. *'Much of what has been learned will be applicable across the working of the health authority' – North Derbyshire. 'Discussions, with others … about progressing the clinical effectiveness agenda, which will be usurped by clinical governance, often include the phrase "what we have learned from the PACE project is …" '* – Walsall.

Key references: Action learning

- *Learning organisations.* The fifth discipline. Senge PM. New York: Doubleday, 1990

Questions to address: Learning the lessons

* Does the agenda for project team (or similar) meetings for members include time to reflect on progress and learning and document the lessons from the work?
* Are facilitation skills available to support the project team?
* Are project team members willing to share mistakes as well as successes? How could they be encouraged?
* Could a project diary help you record key decisions and lessons?
* Are arrangements in place to share the lessons from the work across the organisation?
* Have the lessons from the work informed a strategic approach to promoting effective clinical practice in the organisation?

Managing implementation in the new NHS

The criteria to guide the choice of the 16 projects included the proposals for managing the work as well as the importance of the proposal locally and the evidence-base for the work. The arrangements for the management of the projects varied, with leadership being provided, for example, by clinical consultants, a GP, consultants in public health, a nursing executive director and a medical director. They were supported by a range of project teams and steering/advisory groups. Most projects employed a part-time project manager and/or project co-ordinator.

The detailed work undertaken in the projects has identified three challenges for those leading this type of work in the NHS:

- establishing and maintaining *links* between parallel activities – such as work on standards, audit and education
- ensuring an appropriate *balance* between these activities – and not putting excessive effort into one activity at the expense of others – such as devoting too much time to the creation of standards and insufficient to the delivery of an education and training programme
- ensuring that the separate activities are adequately *aligned* and do not get out of step with others – such as allowing work on guidelines to get ahead of work with patients.

Managing implementation: a project approach

Experience suggests that reliance on separate projects, set up to run alongside the main local systems, to deliver improvements in practice may not be sustainable in the long term. These doubts arise from questions about resources and the subsequent need for mechanisms to sustain change driven from outside the routine systems within organisations. However, implementing change will be an essential element of the new NHS. Local implementation initiatives will need to be planned and executed as part of wider programmes of work and/or as catalytic activities to drive the integration of local systems to support the development of effective health care organisations. Planning such initiatives will require attention to questions about *who* needs to be involved and *what* is intended.

Being clear **who** needs to be involved and their roles

There are four distinct roles:

- *Leading the work.* The complexity of the task emphasises the need to ensure that the 'right' person is identified. Key characteristics of that individual need to include their status locally, their ability to influence others and make connections to cross-departmental and organisational boundaries and their knowledge of both the clinical topic chosen for attention and managing change. *'Leadership of the project by the director of nursing proved essential in influencing key stakeholders on the trust board and in the health authority'* – Chase Farm.

- *Co-ordinating the work.* Virtually all the projects employed someone to 'keep the show together' – a project co-ordinator or a project manager. *'The project manager was a clinical nurse specialist and was a credible source of expertise'* – Wigan and Bolton. Trying to manage the work without such support proved to be difficult. *'A deliberate decision was made not to recruit a project manager to enable us to see whether the project approach could be incorporated with routine, day-to-day work. Possible but difficult is the verdict'* – Walsall.

Selection of the 'right' person to undertake this role is important. It is helpful to ensure that this appointment is made *before* the project plan is agreed, so that the appointee can contribute to the discussions. *'It is not sensible to set targets before key workers are in post – this inhibits their creative input'* – Barnet. Experience has shown the merit of appointing someone with strong local links but one project (Chase Farm) showed that external appointments can work when the project co-ordinator has clinical credibility.

- *Doing the work*. An assessment will be required of the resources likely to be needed – in terms of people, time and materials. Establishing a small project team proved helpful in all the projects. The different aspects of the work will require a range of skills and experience, so care is required to identify the 'right' people – for example, many implementation initiatives require IT support – who will provide this? Building on an existing working group may help speed up the process of creating an effective team. But *'It is important not to rely too heavily on one person, staff move on'* – Chase Farm. As the team is established there may be advantages in involving staff with generic *implementation* skills, i.e. those who have knowledge and experience of implementation strategies (such as individuals from quality assurance teams) to complement local clinicians, who will provide *clinical* skills and knowledge. This approach would allow the learning from initiatives to be easily diffused to future projects by those with implementation skills.

Good team working has been a critical element of all of the projects: it is wise to approach the task without too narrow views of the contributions of individuals – many projects identified 'hidden talents' in the course of their work. *'The people appointed to the key positions of educator and auditor were able to work well unsupervised … and be good advocates for the project'* – South Tyneside. Experience has also shown that it is important to ensure that the roles and objectives for individual members are clear. *'Team building at the beginning would have been useful – to agree an action plan and identify missing links'* – Bradford. There should also be agreed contingency plans in case of staff changes. *'Ensure that all key players in the work are briefing an understudy – invite them to meetings'* – Oxfordshire.

Reflecting the overall focus for the work, there may be a natural inclination to concentrate on clinical staff to lead and undertake the work. Experience has, however, shown that effective teams and groups need to bring together staff with clinical and managerial responsibilities and skills. Managerial responsibilities will include questions about local priorities, questions about resources and questions about sustaining and monitoring the longer-term effectiveness of the services. Managers also bring skills in managing change to the work.

It is helpful to consider where overall responsibility for the separate tasks involved in managing change rests and the scale of the contribution required from clinicians and managers. Figure 2.2 illustrates how the balance – and thus lead responsibility – might be struck for each essential task, but managers and clinicians will have to work together on all these tasks to ensure success.

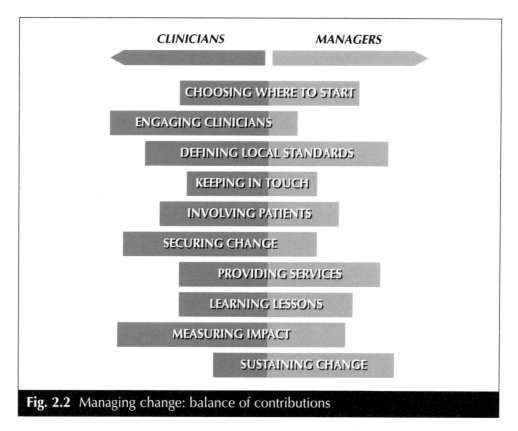

CLINICIANS   MANAGERS

CHOOSING WHERE TO START

ENGAGING CLINICIANS

DEFINING LOCAL STANDARDS

KEEPING IN TOUCH

INVOLVING PATIENTS

SECURING CHANGE

PROVIDING SERVICES

LEARNING LESSONS

MEASURING IMPACT

SUSTAINING CHANGE

Fig. 2.2 Managing change: balance of contributions

- *Providing wider support.* Reflecting the range of interests, all the projects established multi-disciplinary steering and/or senior advisory groups. Membership needs to be considered with care to ensure that all relevant interests are included. However, ways need to be found to progress the work without imposing unrealistic demands on clinicians' time. Key responsibilities of these groups were to: maintain links across organisations, ensure effective communications, ensure that emerging issues were addressed, ensure that senior management was kept in touch with progress and that the lessons from the work were built on.

Being clear about **what** is intended

Experience in the local projects suggests that five aspects need attention.

- *Agreeing realistic objectives and timetable for the work.* Experience in the projects has reinforced earlier views that implementation of changes in clinical practice is a complex task, which takes a significant amount of time and effort. It is wise to ensure a realistic focus for the work. *Barnet intended initially to tackle the management of hypertension – but after the work started and the evidence was reviewed, a narrower focus became sensible, with concentration on older people.*

- *Adopting proven management techniques.* Reflecting the complexity of the work a structured approach to project management will be essential. *Gloucestershire Royal used modified PRINCE methodology with a supporting Gannt chart to facilitate the scheduling of meetings and to keep the separate aspects of the work in step.*

- *Deciding on the tools and techniques to be used.* Research has suggested – and the experience in the local PACE projects demonstrated – that a multi-faceted approach, using a range of intervention techniques (such as local guidelines, educational programmes and audit and feedback), is likely to be effective. The choice should take into account the growing evidence base, such as the reviews undertaken by EPOC.

Work within the Cochrane Effective Practice and the Organisation of Care Review (EPOC) group aims to extend current knowledge about changing clinical behaviour. It would be helpful to review developments in this programme and the emerging lessons from other related works, as new local implementation initiatives are planned.

- *Keeping the work in balance.* Experience has shown the complexity of the work overall and the essential need to ensure that the work is kept in balance. For example, avoid focusing too narrowly on specific tasks, such as agreeing local standards (creating guidelines etc.), when more time may be required to secure change (through the provision of education and training).

- *Monitoring progress.* Experience across the local projects has reaffirmed the need to keep the project plan under review. Flexibility will be important as well as the means to adjust timescales when aspects of the project move ahead more slowly than planned. A link between communications which address messages and information 'outwards' and the collection 'inwards' of information could be helpful.

*Key references and sources. Managing implementation: a project approach*___

- *Cochrane Effective Practice and the Organisation of Care Review Group (EPOC). Closing the gap between research and practice.* Bero L *et al.* BMJ 15 August 1998; 317: 465–268.

– *EPOC module in the Cochrane Library*. Bero L, Grilli R, Grimshaw JM, Mowatt G, Oxman AD (Eds) (1998). Cochrane Effective Practice and Organisation of Care Group. In: The Cochrane Library. Oxford: Update Software, 1998, Issue 4.
– *Organisational change: the key to quality improvement*. Quality in Health Care 1998; 7 (Suppl):S1–S2 [This supplement provides a series of nine important papers about aspects of organisational development]
– *Management of change in health care*. Ferlie E *et al*. The New Public Management in Action. Oxford (1996): Oxford University Press.

Questions to address: Managing implementation: a project approach _____

* Have the aims and objectives for the project been explained to all those likely to be affected by the work? Are the benefits clear?
* Does the plan build on what is known about what works?
* Have you considered the benefits and drawbacks of different strategies for change – such as going for a broad approach covering many practices, or focusing on one initial (pilot) geographic area?
* Is the timetable for the project realistic and flexible?
* What resources are available to support the work?
* Are additional skills required locally to support the work? How will they be secured?
* Have you considered how to balance effort across the ten essential tasks?
* Are arrangements in place to allow the local project team to review systematically progress with the project and adjust the timetable etc., if necessary?

Managing implementation: moving toward a systematic approach

What does the PACE experience mean for the Government's proposals set out in *A First Class Service*?

The questions raised about the viability of local projects to deliver change on the scale that might be required by the products of the National Institute (national service frameworks etc.) strongly suggest that a systems approach is needed. '*We should work to create a well-organised working environment which, through its processes and systems, supports and enables clinicians to deliver first class care*' – Oxfordshire. Evidence from elsewhere has shown that organisational and systems failure contributes to most practice failures. Local arrangements for clinical governance should thus be focused on systems. Clinical governance should place responsibility on organisations to put such systems in place to ensure the delivery of high-quality health care to patients. A growing body of research evidence is now available to guide the development of local organisations.

To meet their responsibility for clinical governance, the PACE experience suggests that local organisations will need to put in place five linked systems.

1. To enable clinical staff to review, routinely, the quality of current practice. Because local information systems are currently mainly driven by contracting requirements, they do not commonly provide adequate detail to enable clinical staff to review the quality of care they deliver. Reliance has traditionally been placed on designing and undertaking one-off audit projects to allow the degree of investigation necessary: a costly process. Action will be required to develop local IT systems to ensure that they embrace clinical data and that they are accessible and usable by clinicians on a continuous basis.

2. To ensure that standards for care can be established. This will require a proactive approach to managing information. These arrangements will need to embrace access to and the use of information. They will need to cover (internal) information about local services, practice and population health as well as access to external sources. A range of external sources will be relevant. Recent developments have enhanced the infrastructure to assure access to research evidence, such as the creation of the Cochrane Library and the NHS Centre for Reviews and Dissemination. In the future access to *national standards* in the light of the work of the proposed National Institute (NICE) and other national bodies may be of growing importance.

3. To ensure that patients are at the centre of work which develops and monitors local standards. This will include arrangements for patients' views and wishes to influence their own care and treatment as well as service and practice developments generally. Experience in the local projects has shown that this is a complex task.

4. To ensure that the implementation of change is managed effectively. Organisations will need to invest in change management skills; such expertise will prevent the waste arising from the non-implementation of needed change to local practice and service provision. The experience from PACE, other similar initiatives and the emerging evidence from research now provides a firm basis on which organisations can build this capability.

5. To support the development of individuals and clinical teams through a systematic approach to education and training. This will need to build on educational theory and evidence from research about how people and teams learn and develop. Arrangements will need to be in place to assess training needs and to determine how those needs will be met. The introduction of arrangements for regular staff appraisal would play an important part in ensuring that local training programmes are appropriately focused. This work will place responsibility on organisations to ensure that staff are able to join in local education and training programmes, without detriment to their clinical responsibilities. A number of hospitals have started to explore ways to restructure arrangements for 'audit days' into 'learning zones', which offer opportunities for multi-disciplinary learning.

Senior leadership should ensure that these systems are effectively inter-connected. A management style which involves all staff and encourages open discussions about and learning from problems will be essential. Systems management will become as important as performance management.

Key references: Organisational development

- *Time for organisational development in health care organisations.* Koeck C. BMJ 1998; 317:1267–8 (7 November)
- *Organisational change: the key to quality improvement.* Quality in Health Care 1998; 7 (Suppl):S1–S2 [This supplement provides a series of important papers about aspects of organisational development]
- *Education methods.* Davis AD *et al.* Changing physician performance: a systematic review of the effect of continuing medical education strategies. JAMA 1995; 274:700–5.

Chapter 3

The local projects

Sixteen local projects were selected in early 1996 and the selection criteria included the need for change locally and the availability of evidence to provide a basis for the work. Subsequently, specific aims and objectives and related project plans were established for individual projects in discussions between the PACE team and each project leader.

The local team had freedom to deploy the grant (£30,000 over the two years) to complement the resources and facilities being allocated locally to support the project. The grant was used in part to cover the costs of staff allocated to the project – such as specialist nurses and/or audit staff – and in part to cover the costs of training sessions (e.g. locum costs), and the production of supporting material (e.g. guidelines and information leaflets for patients).

The 16 projects and the topics selected are listed in Box 1.

Pages 37–116 below review the 16 local projects. For each project, four questions are addressed:

1. *Why was the project set up?* – a brief note about the background to the project.
2. *What was the evidence base for the work?* – notes about the main features of the evidence basis for the work and key references.
3. *What happened?* – a short story about how the work was taken forward.
4. *What changed?* – notes about the data items which were identified to measure the impact of the work and information to illustrate how those measures changed.

This chapter reflects the information which was available when this report went to press, i.e. in December 1998. The original intention was to identify a basket of appropriate measures, to assemble data to allow the impact to be measured and to provide, alongside the information about the projects, some comparisons with the situation elsewhere. In the event it was not possible to meet all those aims, mainly because of problems of securing those data within the timescale of the programme overall. More detailed information about the impact of their work is available from the contacts for the projects listed in the Appendix.

Box 1 The 16 local projects and the topics selected

The care and treatment of **cardiac patients**

- Lambeth, Southwark and Lewisham and King's Healthcare: *cardiac rehabilitation*
- North Derbyshire: *congestive cardiac failure*
- South Tyneside: *the management of stable angina*

The prevention and management of **stroke**

- Barnet: *hypertension in the elderly*
- Gloucestershire Royal: *the management of stroke patients*

The care and treatment of people with **mental health problems**

- Wirral: *family support in schizophrenia*

The **eradication of H. pylori in the management of dyspepsia**

- Bradford
- Bromley
- Walsall

The management of **continence**

- Dudley
- Wigan and Bolton

The care and treatment of **patients predominantly in primary care**

- Dorset: *menorrhagia*
- Royal Berkshire: *leg ulcers*
- Southern Derbyshire: *back pain*

The care of **patients in hospital**

- Chase Farm: *pressure sores*
- Oxfordshire: *post-operative pain control*

Nevertheless, data are available from fifteen projects and, with suitable caution, the information indicates that encouraging changes are being achieved. A further assessment of the impact of the projects would add significantly to future debates about the effectiveness of action to change clinical practice.

THE CARE AND TREATMENT OF CARDIAC PATIENTS

Three projects within the programme focused on elements of cardiac care: cardiac rehabilitation (Lambeth, Southwark and Lewisham and King's Healthcare), congestive cardiac failure (North Derbyshire), and the management of stable angina (South Tyneside).

Lambeth, Southwark and Lewisham and King's Healthcare

Why was the project set up?

In 1995, the health authority launched a major programme of work on clinical effectiveness. An important component of the programme was a work stream called 'Implementing Clinical Effectiveness' (ICE). The work was focused on primary care and on secondary prevention of coronary heart disease. The choice of coronary heart disease as the focus for the ICE programme was a reflection of its local significance as the leading cause of death locally – accounting for about 22 per cent of deaths. It built on the foundations of the cardiac rehabilitation unit at King's College Hospital that had developed a community-based infrastructure and introduced the idea of outreach work. Earlier studies had shown that one issue that required attention was the mismatch between provision of cardiac rehabilitation and local need. The PACE project was designed to tackle this issue.

What was the evidence base for the work?

Pooled data from several studies have shown that cardiac rehabilitation results in a reduction in overall mortality and cardiovascular mortality. Studies have also shown that rehabilitation programmes improve quality of life. It has been estimated that less than 15 per cent of eligible patients in the USA undergo supervised cardiac rehabilitation, and that the proportion is undoubtedly lower in the UK.

Two key recommendations of recent guidelines are that cardiac rehabilitation requires the skills of a range of professionals and that patients should receive a menu-based programme after individual assessments of needs. Cardiac rehabilitation services can be defined as comprehensive, long-term programmes involving medical evaluation, prescribed exercise, cardiac risk factor modification, education and counselling.

Cardiac rehabilitation: key references _____

- NHS Centre for Reviews and Dissemination – University of York. Cardiac rehabilitation. Effective Health Care. August 1997; Vol 4 No 4.

- Agency of Health Care Policy and Research. Cardiac rehabilitation: clinical practice guideline 17.
- AHCPR. US Department of Health and Human Services. Rockville. USA. 1995.
- World Health Organization. Needs and action priorities in cardiac rehabilitation and secondary prevention in patients with coronary heart disease. Copenhagen: WHO Regional Office for Europe. 1993
- Lewin RJP. Adherence to cardiac rehabilitation guidelines: a survey of rehabilitation programmes in the United Kingdom. BMJ. 1998; 316: 1354–1355.

What happened?

The aim of the project was to support patients following discharge after a cardiac event and to achieve this through the work of a cardiac liaison nurse visiting patients at home and working with patients' practices. To support the nurse's work local guidelines were created and a series of practice-based education sessions designed.

The cardiac liaison nurse helped practices to identify patients with coronary heart disease, to help them set up a practice audit and to devise a protocol and suitable documentation. *The outreach approach was deliberately intended to catalyse the practices to undertake the work themselves rather than to do it for them.* Contact with practice managers proved to be particularly helpful.

Choosing where to start was important and the team decided to work incrementally with practices as patients were discharged from hospital – rather than through any expressed interest by practices. This avoided any bias in the early stages of the project towards those committed to the idea of clinical effectiveness. Financial incentives were a part of the work – for example, access to 'health promotion' funds was offered as a reward for the extra work for practices – although some members of the project team believed that it was inappropriate to reward GPs for providing basic good practice.

Personal relationships with practices proved to be the vital trigger to success. The nurse needed to be clear about what was possible for each practice, and for her, to do. Practices were starting from different situations: there was no point in recommending computerised registers if the practice was only using a computer for prescribing. *Relationships within practices were also important:* there was little point trying to solve internal ('political') problems that were out with the project's remit, such as internal lines of communications. The trick seemed to be to work with the key players – which may not necessarily be the GP – and then the rest of the team. *It proved useful to link practices to other existing local organisations, such as the MAAG, and with other local practices. Many practices seemed hermetically sealed from each other, despite the emergence of primary care groups.*

The project faced problems in identifying patients whose care and treatment fell within the new local guidelines. On the one hand, the Patient Administration System (PAS) at King's College Hospital was incomplete because patients were only coded after discharge. On the other hand, using cardiac rehabilitation nurses to check for eligible patients – by walking round the wards at King's College Hospital – was time-consuming. It also proved difficult to set up a process for evaluating the project because the local information systems did not cover the aspects of care and treatment being tackled by the project.

A small multi-disciplinary team co-ordinated the work: the GP/primary care development practitioner at the health authority, the cardiac liaison nurse at King's College Hospital and a public health consultant at the health authority. Good relationships within the team were important. The team reported regularly to senior staff in the main local organisations. Strong support from senior management was demonstrated by the rapid decisions when the (first) cardiac liaison nurse moved on: she was immediately replaced by an experienced ward sister.

Action to involve patients in the project was a particular cause for pride. Not only were traditional methods used – such as developing patient information and patient-held records – but *patients also helped to define the scope of the project and its development.* Four focus groups of service users were involved (older people, women, men and people from the local Asian community). They have taught clinicians and practices about what was 'effective' from a patient's point of view and made a number of practical – and inexpensive – recommendations. For example, a focus group described how '*the month following discharge was frightening for patients with services sometimes failing them*'. The clinical liaison nurse was able to fill this gap. Other recommendations for good practice included the supply of information, the style of consultations (being treated with respect and dignity) and practice management issues (no telephone interruptions, clear mechanisms for receiving and understanding test results, different lengths of appointments). *Patients have proved to be important change agents.*

Many of the changes achieved by the project will continue – because they have already become an integral part of the provision of care. In addition, the practice-based education sessions and computer-based methods for identifying populations will be maintained. Following training by the cardiac liaison nurse, the visits to patients have already been devolved to local health visitors and district nurses. Plans are already well advanced to use the learning from the project in work on mental health services – the next topic in the ICE programme. Practice visits and user educational initiatives will feature strongly in the work.

What changed?

Because of the absence of relevant routine information the evaluation of this project was a qualitative examination focused on aspects of the work with patients, with practices and the related educational initiative.

To assess the reactions of *patients* to the home visits by community nurses a questionnaire was circulated to a small group (40) of patients who had been seen by the nurse. Three-quarters of the questionnaire were returned. The overall response from patients was positive:

- 69 per cent said the visits made them feel better, as did a similar proportion of relatives
- 83 per cent of recipients found the visits useful.

Points made by the patients included: '*You need a district nurse to help you have a bit of peace of mind when the patient comes home*' and '*At the time I was living alone and these visits were very welcome*'. There were however some areas where the nurse did not discuss important issues with patients such as about drugs or diet. This approach has been integrated into the work of local district nurses.

The work with *practices* centred on visits by the cardiac outreach nurse and involved 19 practices and each practice was visited about seven times. Reports from the visits showed significant progress in encouraging the adoption of audit and the development of local protocols. Changes were noted in all the practices involved; examples include the establishment of practice-based exercise classes, the organisation of 'healthy walks' and a practice-based support group. Some practices were for the first time able to identify a cardiac population and therefore target interventions to them. Practice nurses were the most enthusiastic participants in the work and they achieved significant improvements in care even when there was virtually no GP input. The primary care audit (MARG) evaluation suggested that more change would have resulted if the visits had engaged more GPs.

The *educational initiative* was designed to explore whether users' definition of effectiveness could influence practice. Focus groups of patients were convened and delegates from them subsequently met with GPs and nurses. Evaluation showed that although 83 per cent of the clinicians found the meetings useful, 43 per cent also said they gained little. Nonetheless, a review at six months showed that all the recommendations had been adopted to some extent. Eight per cent of participants were offering patients more information about side-effects, 60 per cent had begun offering appointments of different lengths, 53 per cent were giving more information about investigation results and 60 per cent focusing information on what the patient most wanted to know.

North Derbyshire

Why was the project set up?

Widespread concern expressed locally by GPs about standards of care was the main catalyst for the project proposal. The project focused on improving the investigation and management of patients with congestive heart failure. It was attractive because it involved so many disciplines and fitted into the *Health of the Nation* strategy: it was bound to have wide-ranging impact. The specific aims were to increase prescribing of ACE inhibitors and to develop open access echocardiography.

What was the evidence base for the work?

Heart failure is a life threatening condition that affects between 0.4 per cent and 2.0 per cent of the general population and up to 10 per cent of elderly subjects in the UK. The condition is also responsible for around 5 per cent of all admissions to hospital each year and costs the National Health Service almost £360 million a year. Measures of impairment of quality of life identify heart failure as causing greater impairment than other common conditions such as diabetes, arthritis, chronic lung problems or angina.

There is overwhelming evidence from controlled trials to suggest that patients with heart failure would benefit from treatment with ACE inhibitors. There is also good evidence that the use of ACE inhibitors reduces the rate of hospitalisation for heart failure by approximately 30 per cent, and reduces the re-admission rate by at least 5 per cent. Evidence also suggests that reductions in mortality and morbidity can be achieved through raising awareness and education on appropriate investigation and treatment.

Congestive cardiac failure: key references _____

- Garg R, Yusuf S. ACE collaboration group. JAMA 1995;273(18): 1450–56
- Rector TS. ACE inhibitors and quality of life. Coronary Artery Disease 1995; 6(4):310–14.
- Francis CM *et al*. Open access echocardiography in the management of heart failure in the community. BMJ 1995; 310: 634–36.
- ATLAS Trial. Assessment of Treatment with Lisinopril and Survival. 47th Annual American College of Cardiology (ACC) Scientific Session. Atlanta GA, USA. 1998.

What happened?

Three main streams formed the work programme. First, to support GPs to undertake an audit of their current practice and identify patients whose current treatment merited review. Second, to provide an education programme about congestive heart failure. Third, to provide better access to diagnostic echocardiography in the five local acute hospitals. *The overall emphasis was on information about the condition and treatment **not** on the rigid application of strict guidelines.*

One of the first tasks was to produce and distribute to practices an information pack containing advice about the project, the research evidence, the proposed audit and material about use of ACE inhibitors and cost benefit analysis. This was followed up by an initial programme of formal GP educational meetings. These sessions focused on the project, echocardiography as a diagnostic tool and the proposed audit. The meetings were well attended. A second series of sessions in 1998 focused on open-access services, the re-audit, and management of those patients with heart failure not confirmed by echocardiography. These sessions were complemented by a practice nurse study day. As with other strands of the work, this was an example of the way in which *the project team worked through existing systems*. The sessions were arranged as part of an annual GP education programme, through the University of Sheffield and had PGEA approval.

A pilot with three GP practices provided the test-bed before the audit guide was offered to other practices. The subsequent audit was completed in 48 (78 per cent) practices. The re-audit (in 80 per cent of practices) was undertaken 15–24 months later. Factors which secured the high level of participation included the pre-existing strong culture of primary care audit in North Derbyshire; the active invitation through the primary care quality group to all practices to take part in the audit; local interest in a 'quality of life' survey and the supporting education programme. Practices were offered either a financial payment for doing the audit themselves or the services of an audit nurse.

Information booklets for patients and carers were distributed through practices, pharmacies and local centres. The CHC was also involved in pilots of the quality of life survey and this patient and public involvement strand of the work has built on a good on-going relationship with the CHC.

Ensuring that initiatives to change clinical practice were matched by funding for, and changes to, service levels and configuration was a major objective from the outset. Increased referral activity was catered for by ensuring access to echocardiography at most of the local provider units to manage congestive cardiac failure.

Features of the way in which the project was set up and maintained contributed to its success. The project leader, a consultant in public health and an ex-GP, was well known to and respected by GPs. The project officer had strong local links and could build on existing relationships. The team attended local meetings to report on progress and enlist help and support. The project officer was a central contact point, and while not full time, benefited from support from conscientious secretarial staff. A wider project group included representatives from primary and secondary care and the health authority.

The team consistently *focused on ways to work within existing networks*, such as encouraging locality managers to reinforce the work during practice visits. *Implementation has been tackled in a staged manner*, allowing sufficient time for each activity to be incorporated before the next one was introduced. *Communication both within the team and to stakeholders has been regular and focused.* A project timetable has been helpful with regular meetings and quarterly newsletters.

It was not all plain sailing and inevitably some unexpected challenges arose. The 'purchaser/provider' system meant difficulties in some localities in obtaining support for the open access developments. More time to visit practices and explain the work on a more regular basis would also have been beneficial, as would earlier involvement of practice nurses.

Despite concerns locally that the project might be seen as separate from the mainstream work of organisations, recent events have been *encouraging for sustaining and generalising from the changes which have been achieved.* Local open-access echocardiography services will continue. Visits from the pharmaceutical adviser to practices for prescribing reviews will sustain the message and use, and costs of ACE inhibitors and loop diuretics will continue to be monitored.

The project has involved a broader approach to primary care teams in this type of development: not just GPs but also practice managers, practice nurses and – for the first time – community pharmacists. *The seeds have been sown for future development work and the way in which clinicians should be involved in, for example, primary care groups. The learning within the project group itself will be of considerable value for future work in other clinical topics.*

What changed?

Encouraging the use of echocardiography in patients with suspected heart failure was expected to increase the prescription of ACE inhibitors and decrease inappropriate prescribing of loop diuretics. ACE inhibitors are known to reduce mortality in heart failure. It was expected that adequate treatment of the condition would also lead to reduced hospital admissions and a reduction in re-admissions. The impact on length of stay was also monitored.

The measures for this project were:

- *Prescribing (PACT) data*   *Loop diuretics*
                                    Loop compound diuretics
                                    ACE inhibitors
- *Diagnostic testing*   *ECHO cardiographic referrals*
- *Referral activity*   *Appropriateness of referral*
- *Inpatient activity*   *Admissions for heart failure*
                                    Re-admissions for heart failure
                                    Length of stay for heart failure
                                    Hospital deaths from heart failure

Figures 3.1–3.4 provide information related to these measures which was available in November 1998.

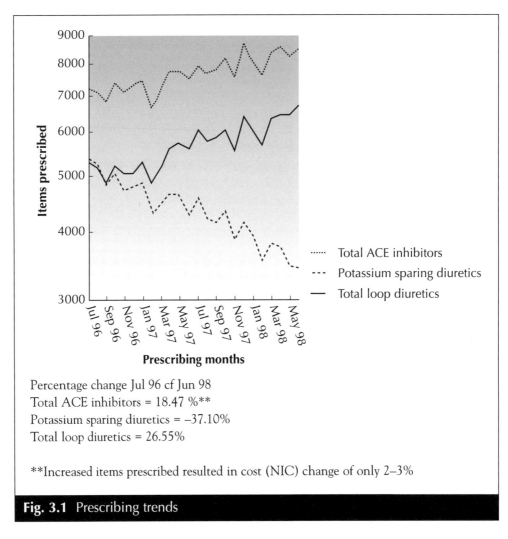

Percentage change Jul 96 cf Jun 98
Total ACE inhibitors = 18.47 %**
Potassium sparing diuretics = −37.10%
Total loop diuretics = 26.55%

**Increased items prescribed resulted in cost (NIC) change of only 2–3%

Fig. 3.1 Prescribing trends

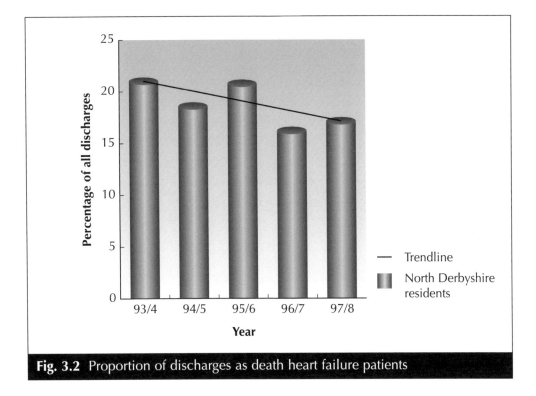

Fig. 3.2 Proportion of discharges as death heart failure patients

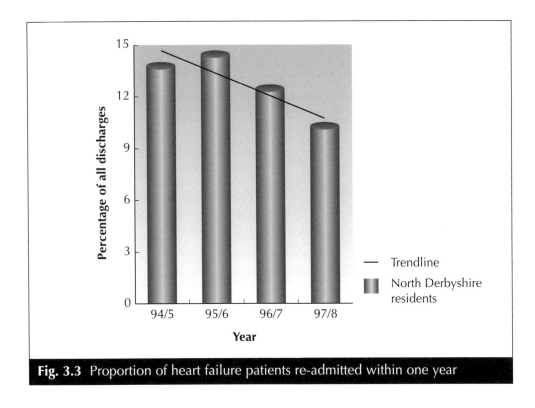

Fig. 3.3 Proportion of heart failure patients re-admitted within one year

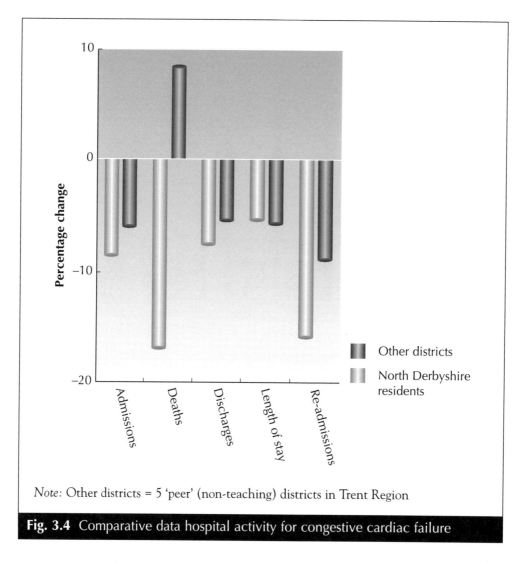

Note: Other districts = 5 'peer' (non-teaching) districts in Trent Region

Fig. 3.4 Comparative data hospital activity for congestive cardiac failure

South Tyneside

Why was the project set up?

A local report in 1994 had demonstrated that South Tyneside had one of the highest mortalities from ischaemic heart disease in England; over 30 per cent of acute medical admissions were related to ischaemic heart disease. Other work had shown that the standard of care provided to patients compared unfavourably with neighbouring districts. Following these studies a series of joint audit projects were undertaken to examine the management of patient care in the district and identify the scope for improvement. The overall aim of this project was to improve the care provided to patients with ischaemic heart disease and build on local goodwill established by many of the project team during the earlier work.

What was the evidence base for the work?

People with stable angina are at increased risk of heart attack and death. Targeting this group with effective treatments is an important component of a coronary heart strategy. Other important elements in the treatment of stable angina include the use of low dose aspirin, lipid lowering therapies and other risk factor management either as primary treatment or as an adjunct to invasive procedures.

Stable angina: key references _____

- NHS Centre for Reviews and Dissemination – University of York. Management of stable angina. Effective Health Care. October 1997; Vol 3 No 5.
- Scandinavian Simvastatin Survival Study Group. Randomised trial of cholesterol lowering in 4444 patients with coronary heart disease: the Scandinavian Simvastatin Survival Study (4S). Lancet 1994; 344: 1383–9.
- Shepherd *et al*. Prevention of coronary heart disease with Pravastatin in men with hyper-cholesterolaemia (WOSCOPs). NEJM 1995; 333: 1301–7.

What happened?

The plan was to improve the quality of patient care through the delivery of a package of audit and educational activities to support the use of a locally produced guideline for the management of chronic stable angina in primary and secondary care. The project was led by a local consultant physician within a multi-disciplinary project team. From the outset, *effort was devoted to building up a network of professional interest and support for the project's aims.* The provision locally of an open access exercise ECG testing was an added incentive for primary care involvement.

A local guideline pack was created for use in primary and secondary care. This work took as a starting point work on chronic stable angina undertaken by the North of England Evidence-Based Guidelines Development Project. Particular attention was paid to creating material that was concise, credible and user-friendly: *presentation was deemed as important as content.* The launch of the local guideline was followed by an educational programme tailored to the needs of individuals. This involved the creation of '*study guide workbooks*' which allowed participants to monitor their own learning. This programme was targeted at practice nurses, practice managers, as well as staff in the local NHS trust staff, GPs and community pharmacists. The workbooks were approved by the University of Northumbria and accredited for educational purposes. The project team was able to identify barriers and opportunities for further educational initiatives as they managed and delivered the educational programme.

Local practice audits were programmed for six months after the local educational sessions. Reporting of the results of the audits was *designed as a further learning exercise* – to highlight shortcomings within management and treatment of angina. Initially the emphasis was on practice-related data but as the project evolved league tables were developed and PACE Charter Marks set in relation to project targets.

Alongside the work with primary care teams, the project team believed that *patients could and should be agents for change* and saw the potential of a patient-held record as an important means of patient empowerment. A patient focus group helped to refine the record as well as reinforce messages to clinicians. There are plans to evaluate the impact of the patient-held record. The messages to patients have also been well publicised through local newsletters and the media.

Regular project team meetings have allowed the team to review progress, identify lessons learned and consider solutions to emerging problems. However, despite the multi-disciplinary teamwork, a small group of people undertook most of the work and some team members felt less involved. While there were opportunities for members of the team to develop new skills, with hindsight more could have been done to *define the skill-mix required* prior to the launch of the project. For example, two key appointments brought educational and audit expertise to the project team – but only after the project had been going for some time. Similarly, the process of keeping all those affected by the project up to date with progress and problems could have been handled better if the creation of a communications strategy had been an early task for the project team. *A key message was that a project like this is 80 per cent planning and 20 per cent operational.*

The *need for flexibility* became evident as the project was taken forward and some of the more ambitious aspects delayed, for example work on lifestyle advice and a patient satisfaction survey. This allowed the team to concentrate on maintaining the education programme for clinicians. The project team were sensitive to the pressures on primary care teams and *adopted an incremental approach* – with careful staging of the work on guidelines, education, audit and the introduction of the patient-held record.

One of the main stumbling blocks was the limited support from the trust and health authority – a consequence of senior staff changes. This lack of enthusiasm was not mirrored in primary care, where the project team were well received. Discussions are continuing to institutionalise the improvements in clinical practice and the lessons learned locally during the project. An important aspect of this could be the *introduction of active management of IHD services* – as part of new arrangements for clinical governance – involving a partnership between the health authority, primary care groups and cardiac services within the NHS trust.

What changed?

A combination of audit and routine data was used to assess the impact on clinical practice both in primary care and in secondary care. Mortality rates for coronary heart disease have been falling in South Tyneside. It will take several years to determine the effect of the introduction of the guidelines. Similarly, there has been no demonstrable difference in aspirin prescribing in South Tyneside and Gateshead. Both districts had undertaken projects prior to PACE directed at increasing aspirin prescribing.

The measures for the project were:

- *Referral activity*   *Open access ECG*
  Exercise ECGs
  Myo scans
  Lipids

- *Prescribing data*   *Aspirin (75mg and 300 mg)*#*
  Oral nitrate*#
  Beta-blockers*# (Atenolol & propranolol as a proportion of total beta-blockers)

*PACT data, #Inpatient hospital prescribing

There has been a small but definite increase in beta-blocker prescribing as a result of the project. There has also been a definite increase in aspirin, oral nitrate and beta-blocker prescribing in inpatient hospital prescribing in the year following the introduction of the guidelines.

Figures 3.5–3.9 provide information related to these measures which was available in November 1998.

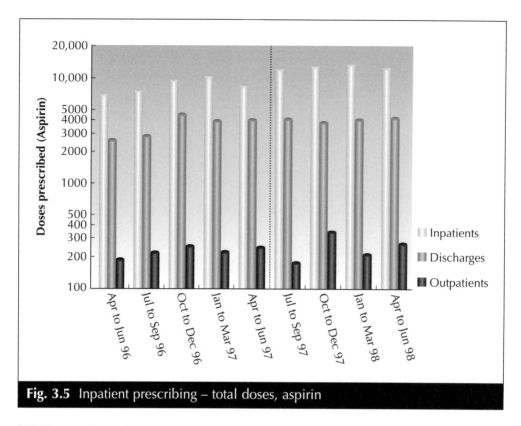

Fig. 3.5   Inpatient prescribing – total doses, aspirin

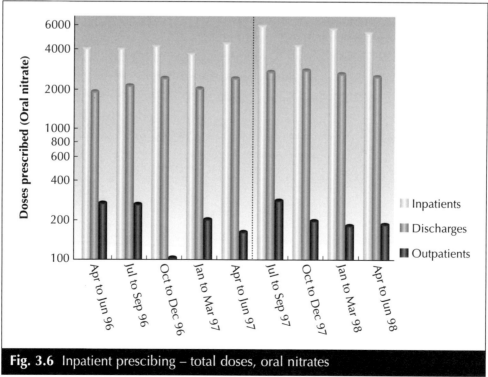

Fig. 3.6   Inpatient prescibing – total doses, oral nitrates

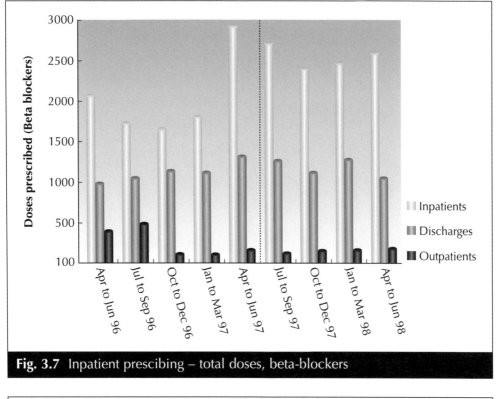

Fig. 3.7 Inpatient prescibing – total doses, beta-blockers

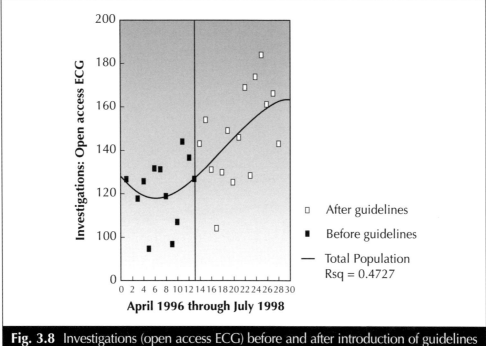

Fig. 3.8 Investigations (open access ECG) before and after introduction of guidelines

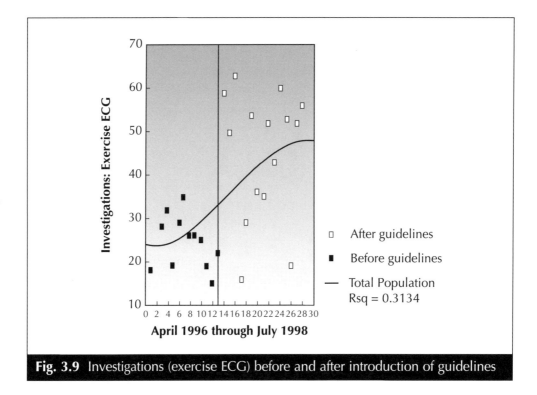

Fig. 3.9 Investigations (exercise ECG) before and after introduction of guidelines

THE PREVENTION AND MANAGEMENT OF STROKE

Two projects within the programme related to the prevention and management of stroke and were focused on the management of hypertension in the elderly (Barnet) and the management of stroke patients in hospital (Gloucestershire Royal).

Barnet

Why was the project set up?

The project was set up to address a key *Health of the Nation* objective, the reduction of stroke in the 65–74 year age group. It aimed to develop a collaborative approach to stroke prevention in primary care in Barnet, an outer North London health authority district. In particular to:

- build on existing locally obtained data about GP attitudes and practice relating to stroke prevention
- undertake additional audit on the detection and management of stroke risk factors and disseminate results of audits
- provide information and research evidence within the context of an educational programme
- work with local stakeholders on strategies to improve the management of stroke risk factors in primary care.

What was the evidence base for the work?

Hypertension (high blood pressure) is the major risk factor for stroke. National and local surveys indicate that it is inadequately detected and treated, particularly in older people, even though trial evidence shows that treatment of the elderly is highly effective. Timely and adequate control of hypertension has been shown to reduce the risk of stroke by at least a third. Despite the emerging evidence, a 1993 survey of Barnet GPs had shown that they were less likely to initiate treatment at a given level of blood pressure in older than in younger patients. An audit of stroke cases in Barnet during 1995 showed deficiencies in blood pressure recording prior to the occurrence of stroke.

Control of blood pressure is particularly important in the presence of other risk factors (e.g. smoking, high cholesterol, diabetes and end-organ damage or clinical cardiovascular disease) and these factors also need to be addressed. Randomised controlled trials have also shown the value of aspirin in patients with previous strokes or TIAs (transient ischaemic attacks) and anticoagulation in atrial fibrillation in appropriately selected patients.

Stroke prevention (hypertension in the elderly): key references _____

- L Hansson *et al*. Effects of intensive blood pressure lowering and low dose aspirin in patients with hypertension: principal results of the Hypertension Optimal Treatment (HOT) randomised trial. Lancet 1998; 351:1755–1762
- Collins *et al*. Benefits of lowering BP in the general population: review of 14 randomised trials of antihypertensives. Lancet 1990; 335:827–38
- Sanderson S. Hypertension in the elderly: pressure to treat? Health Trends 1996; 28(4)
- The sixth report of the Joint National Committee on prevention, detection, evaluation, and treatment of high blood pressure. Arch Intern Med. 1997; Nov 24; 157(21):2413–46

What happened?

The initial project proposal was designed to address primary and secondary stroke prevention but it was decided early on to concentrate on the management of hypertension in the context of other risk factors and to target in particular older patients (over 60s). *This highlights a tension which many projects faced: how to balance work on a narrower, perhaps more feasible, target with wider concerns.*

The project team consisted of two part-time local primary care practitioners, a GP and – later – a practice nurse, supported by a doctor and a research officer from the public health department. Other members of the public health department worked on an *ad hoc* basis, including a pharmaceutical adviser and public health trainees.

Initially the project fell behind the planned timetable because of unforeseeable staff factors including illness, bereavement and personnel changes. It was hard for the project team to overcome these difficulties. However, the GP and the project nurse facilitator were able to secure accreditation for their educational work and target a significant proportion of practices. Their creativity and experience enabled them to steer the project. The project became *more evolutionary and incremental than deadline-focused: the real world of implementation.*

The project team held to its model of multi-disciplinary involvement throughout: project meetings were frequent as well as meetings with an advisory/steering group consisting of other GPs, chair of the LMC, consultant physicians, academics, Stroke Association and CHC representatives. In addition contacts were made with the GP tutors, local education board, MAAG and prescribing committee. The project was able to influence the agenda of these groups. Material developed by the project team included: a GP education pack; a GP case study exercise; hypertension audit tools; posters; and there are plans to pilot a patient-held record.

The plan included the development of stroke prevention or hypertension guidelines. Discussion at the initial advisory group meeting produced differing views about the development of guidelines: ranging from the adoption of a single threshold for intervention to a complex, preferably computerised, risk stratification approach. Difficulties in maintaining a consistent group meant the process of guideline development was not ideal. Draft guidelines were presented to the advisory group but were rejected as being too long and as little more than an amalgamation of existing guidelines. The pilot audit had shown that the British Hypertension Society Guidelines were being used in the majority of practices but that local guidelines would be valued. The educational visits to GPs were used to consult GPs on this question. As part of the pack the recently amended British Hypertension Society guidelines are presented together with both the New Zealand risk tables and the risk stratification tool published in the US guidelines. GPs have found the document to be of particularly useful in clinical practice.

Over the course of the project, national and international guidelines were moving away from the threshold approach to intervention towards multiple risk factor assessment and stratification. The educational materials were modified to reflect this change. A programme of accredited educational events was set up for GPs, practice nurses and pharmacists. Different types of educational events helped to get the message across – *the evidence shows that it is best to tailor the approach to the target audience*. The main method of involving GPs was outreach visits: tutorials on research evidence and implementation. PGEA approval was given for the visit plus a subsequent case study. Follow-up visits to practice nurses were undertaken by the nurse facilitator. In conjunction with the Barnet Primary Care Education and Development Board, an innovative modular hypertension course was devised for practice nurses. Two courses have been held so far.

GPs were invited to audit the management of hypertension among people aged over 60 within their practice: many were unable to complete the task. Resource constraints (time and support) and less than perfect IT systems were to blame. However, after the results of the audit were shared with GPs, many others have shown a growing interest in the project. Practice nurses were asked to do a similar audit as part of the hypertension course. A different approach to audit is being tried following the GP visits involving case studies on high-risk patients.

The project team were keen to develop ways of providing information to patients. In collaboration with the local Stroke Association and CHC an information leaflet and patient-held record have been developed. Practice nurses attending the hypertension course will undertake a pilot project using the record cards. Another way of ensuring the message got through was to link with other events and campaigns: for example, promotional activities (including blood pressure screening sessions) were timed to coincide with National Stroke Weeks.

Looking to the future: the practice visits and the practice nurse hypertension course will continue. The MAAG is planning to incorporate audit of stroke risk factor management into its programme and primary stroke prevention work is a key aspect of the local health improvement programme. The appointment of a co-ordinator to work on secondary prevention of stroke is under consideration. Finally, the lessons learned from the PACE project will be invaluable in developing work with GPs to deliver other clinical effectiveness packages.

What changed?

The project built on the findings from a local survey undertaken by the Royal Free Hospital School of Medicine, which identified insufficient awareness of the need for good blood pressure control in the elderly. There was also evidence from a retrospective audit of prior management of stroke cases to suggest that there were deficiencies in standards of documentation. As part of the project, two main audits were undertaken: an audit of management in patients over 60 and a new stroke risk stratification exercise on 20 patients aged over 60 in each practice.

Prescription data for antihypertensive agents provide a crude indicator of the management of hypertension during the time of the project (see Fig. 3.10). ACE inhibitors are used for purposes other than antihypertensive therapy (e.g. cardiac failure) and as such are only a crude indicator.

Gloucestershire Royal

Why was the project set up?

A multi-disciplinary Stroke Steering Group has been well established in Gloucester for several years. The project was proposed as a direct consequence of a multi-disciplinary audit of the management and outcomes of over 350 stroke patients undertaken in 1995. The audit demonstrated the lack of systematic co-ordination of care for patients and considerable variability in clinical practice.

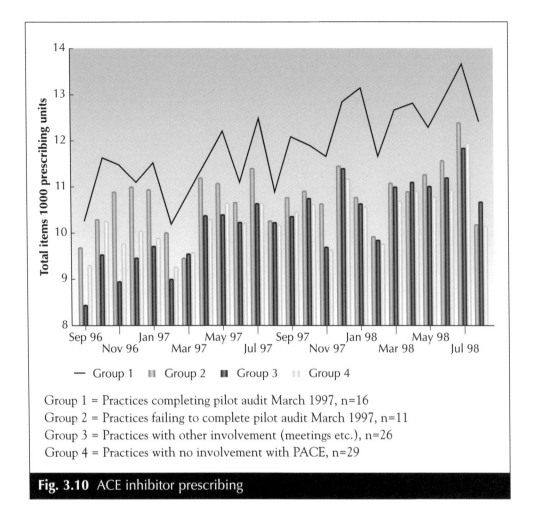

Group 1 = Practices completing pilot audit March 1997, n=16
Group 2 = Practices failing to complete pilot audit March 1997, n=11
Group 3 = Practices with other involvement (meetings etc.), n=26
Group 4 = Practices with no involvement with PACE, n=29

Fig. 3.10 ACE inhibitor prescribing

What was the evidence base for the work?

Stroke is a common disabling and life-threatening condition. Epidemiological studies have indicated that approximately two people in every thousand are admitted to hospital with stroke each year. Approximately 20 per cent of patients die within a month of their first stroke and 35 per cent of the survivors are dependent at six months.

Recent evidence indicates that organised inpatient (stroke unit) care results in long-term reductions in death, dependency and the need for institutional care. The evidence also suggests that the important characteristics of care are the provision of co-ordinated multi-disciplinary rehabilitation, staff specialisation in stroke or rehabilitation and improved education and training.

The management of stroke: key reference _____

• Stroke unit trialists' collaboration. Collaborative review of randomised trials of organised inpatient (stroke unit) care after stroke. BMJ 1997; 314:1151–9

What happened?

Better post-stroke care was the aim for the project and the mechanism to deliver this was the development of an 'integrated care pathway' for acute care and rehabilitation. This approach offered a potentially valuable means for bringing together the different contributions of all health care professionals and acting as a focus for multi-disciplinary working.

A multi-disciplinary project team was established comprising members of the original steering group and also included the newly appointed stroke case manager and care pathway co-ordinator. Initially the project needed to develop a shared understanding of care pathways prior to making their own contributions to the emerging stroke care pathway. An initial reluctance to share experiences stemmed from lack of knowledge and experience of care pathways as well as the perception that professional practice was being critically reviewed, and the different levels of research evidence to support practice in some of the professions. However, enthusiasm increased once the integrated care pathway was produced in a practical form. It was at this point that all staff were able to gain a real understanding of the care pathway and how it would benefit their practice in providing patient care.

Members of the project team were responsible for the training of colleagues in the use and completion of the new documentation accompanying the care pathway – prior to a three-month pilot period. Review of the pilot resulted in a number of modifications. A pro-forma has since been developed for the weekly multi-disciplinary team meeting which includes the projection of measurable goals and outcomes for patients. Arrangements are also being put in place to ensure that the evidence base for the pathway is updated: changes have already been made to incorporate recent evidence about the use of drug pyrimidole.

A project board led by an executive director of the trust provided leadership and direction for the project: membership included a consultant in elderly care, the general manager for medicine and elderly care, the chair of the audit committee, a consultant in community medicine, the care pathway co-ordinator and project manager. The project was managed using modified PRinCE methodology. A Gannt chart was created to form the detailed project plan and to provide a framework for scheduling the timing of the project board meetings thus enabling key decisions and progress.

A communication strategy was devised to keep staff informed about the progress and to consult with them as the pathway was being developed. Presentations and discussions within the medical directorate were arranged as well as contributions to the individual disciplines' regular meetings. The project achieved high profile within the trust and members of the team presented reports on the progress to the trust board as well as the public via, for example, the trust, also attended by the CHC and local councillors. Training for staff was provided to explain the nature and purpose of integrated care pathways. In addition, support in the use of the new documentation was provided by the care pathway co-ordinator and stroke case manager.

As part of the project, a patient and carer support group has been set up by the rehabilitation clinical psychologist and the stroke case manager. This has led to the use of a new clinical psychology assessment framework to enable nursing staff to identify which patients and/or carers would benefit most from support. The pathway has contributed to the reorganisation of the services, which has in turn led to a streamlined referral process and the designation of stroke beds. The stroke care pathway also serves as a template for further care pathways. Presently, 22 care pathways are under development and implementation, including fractured neck of femur, breast surgery, pneumonia, tonsillectomy and cystoscopy. The experience of this project suggests that success will be more likely if the 'right' members of staff are included in the project team: a structured approach is adopted to achieve objectives and responses from colleagues are heeded. Building on progress so far, the trust has been recruited into two multi-centre clinical trials and two nationally recognised audits.

What changed?

Changes in the management of stroke at Gloucestershire Royal included the introduction of a unified patient record, the development of an integrated care pathway and the appointment of a stroke co-ordinator.

Four audits were undertaken to measure the impact of change during the course of the two-year project. The four stages of the evaluation comprised baseline, transitional, pre-implementation and post-change audits. Results from the audit were analysed against agreed aspects of quality:

- *Accessibility – speed of team assessment and commencement of investigations*
- *Effectiveness – conformance to care pathways and analysis of variance*
- *Efficacy – achieving the right results.*

Overall the audit results show an increase in the frequency of inpatients returning to their original address – up from 40 per cent to 50 per cent. In addition, the length of stay has been reduced from 60 days (in 1995) to 33 days (1997) for 80 per cent of the sample to be discharged.

Figures 3.11–3.13 provide additional detail of changes over the duration of the project.

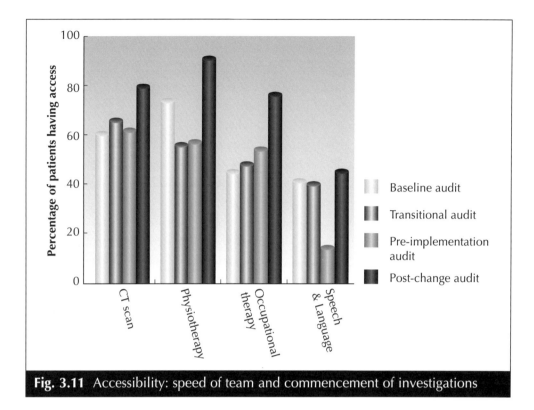

Fig. 3.11 Accessibility: speed of team and commencement of investigations

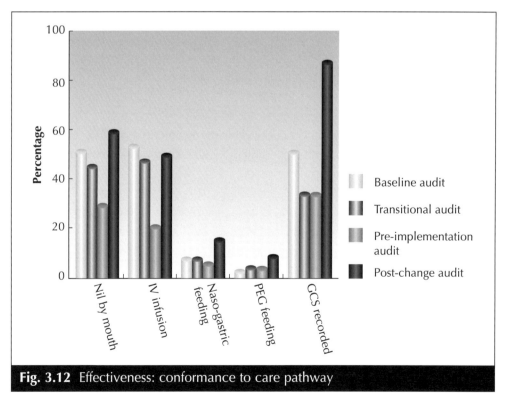

Fig. 3.12 Effectiveness: conformance to care pathway

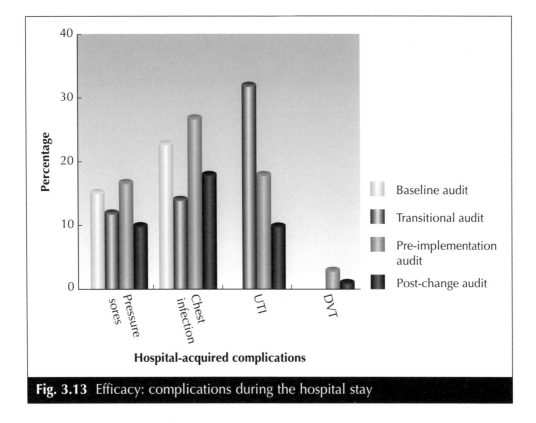

Fig. 3.13 Efficacy: complications during the hospital stay

THE CARE AND TREATMENT OF PEOPLE WITH MENTAL HEALTH PROBLEMS

One project focused on the provision of family therapy in schizophrenia (Wirral).

Wirral

Why was the project set up?

Wirral Health Authority and Wirral Social Services Department completed a comprehensive review of mental health services in September 1995. The statutory agencies committed themselves to addressing, in partnership with relevant voluntary organisations, a number of areas for development. One aspect of the review identified as a target group the most seriously mentally ill and their families. The project was set up to respond to this aspect of the review.

What was the evidence for the work?

Schizophrenia is a relatively common form of psychotic disorder (severe mental illness). Its life time prevalence is nearly 1 per cent and its annual incidence is around 10–15 per 100,000. The average general practitioner cares for 10–20 schizophrenic patients, depending on social circumstances and location.

A recent systematic review of the effects of family psychosocial interventions concluded that families may expect the member with schizophrenia to relapse less and to be in hospital less. The review also found that intervention encouraged compliance with medication and may help people stay in employment. Psychosocial interventions are normally provided as part of a wider treatment package, including routine drug treatment. The aims of the intervention are to:

- improve the family's knowledge and understanding of schizophrenia
- improve service users' adherence to treatment
- improve carers' recognition of signs of relapse
- enhance coping strategies for dealing with difficult and disruptive behaviour
- improve the quality of life of service users and carers.

Family support in schizophrenia: key references

- Mari JJ, Streiner D. Family intervention for schizophrenia. (Cochrane Review) In: The Cochrane Library, Issue 2. Oxford: Update Software; 1998. Updated quarterly.

- Dixon L, Lehman A. Family interventions for schizophrenia. Schizophrenia Bulletin 1995; 21(4):631–43.
- Department of Health. Report of a clinical standards advisory group on schizophrenia. Vol 1. London: HMSO, 1995.
- Huxley P. Making More Space. The unique and vital contribution of the family support worker. The University of Manchester and Making Space.

What happened?

The employment of a family support worker through a voluntary sector organisation – 'Making Space' – was the focus for this project. The post was set in the multi-disciplinary community mental health team to provide dedicated support to carers. Integration was favoured over developing a stand-alone service.

Following the appointment of the family support worker, the project team decided that an incremental approach was essential – there was a risk that the single family support worker would be overwhelmed by referrals. A phased introduction of the service was therefore planned, with referrals controlled by the pace at which general practices were involved. *This phased approach made it possible to measure demand and referral characteristics of patients and carers. This process did, however, cause some frustration because of the family support worker's time was not fully occupied by the project: other activities were undertaken until a full caseload was achieved.*

The appointment of the family support worker was supported by *information packs* which were designed to describe the service and routes of referral. A *range of education and training activities were also arranged to raise awareness of the needs of carers and the benefits of the family support worker approach.* These included: work with users and carers, education sessions about the role of the family support worker, care management discussions involving the family support worker and carers to expose the team to carers' views.

One major problem was that the service was not fully utilised because of the traditional view that the community psychiatric nurse was *the* member of the team who should look after the user-carer interface. There was a view that a dedicated carer support worker might damage the professional-client relationship. *These difficulties stimulated useful thinking about the appropriateness of other members of the team acting as gate-keepers to services for the family.* These discussions led the project team to decide that the family support worker should select clients as an alternative to a formal referral process. Meanwhile, the community psychiatric nurses were involved in a study to identify the needs of all known local sufferers of schizophrenia. *The parallel processes – the selection approach of the family support worker and the referrals to community psychiatric nurses – became seen as a comprehensive system.*

The discussions that the family support worker role provoked enabled the community mental health team *to clarify roles and responsibilities – while retaining separate functions – and to ensure that needs were met.* Staff worries about who would join the team were overcome by *involving them in discussions* on models of working. Joint training was difficult to manage because different agencies were responsible for different members of the teams – but these difficulties were not allowed to prevent the provision of suitable training.

The role of the voluntary sector was a distinctive feature of this project. Some staff felt that there was a risk that voluntary sector staff within the community mental health team might disrupt established monitoring arrangements and, perhaps, standards of care, *but the overall perception was favourable.* Multi-agency and multi-professional approaches resulted in a *greater understanding of the need for a more holistic approach to care delivery.* Local consultant psychiatrists helped to legitimise the approach by recommending the extension of the employment of additional family support workers within the three other existing community mental health teams.

Managing the project was only one part of a wider approach which followed the mental health services review. The project was not accorded special status and the work was integrated with other initiatives and maintained at an operational level. There was a clear expectation that the NHS worked closely with Making Space and thus develop arrangements for jointly managing this type of initiative.

The inter-professional tensions which arose during the project were, in the end, seen as a positive contribution to client care. *The different training, educational and philosophical beliefs of the team members added to the quality of options for care.* The experiences of integrating the family support worker into the work of the community mental health team also yielded useful lessons for the future. Experience in the project has shown that *the views of carers* should be more readily taken as a valid component in assessments of clients' mental health status and care needs – and that individual carers merit support for their own needs.

In the field of mental health, staff often feel threatened by audits and other management initiatives: defensiveness to new ideas is not surprising. Attempts to change staff through coercion will not work. *However, long-term exposure to alternatives does lead to changes: stamina and persistence are essential. This project validates 'slow exposure' as a valid change agent.*

What changed?

Wirral developed a monitoring tool for their local evaluation adapted from the 'active caseload sheet' originally developed by Making Space. Quantitative information arising from the caseload monitoring sheets was embellished by more qualitative information provided by the family support worker herself.

The evidence base for family intervention for schizophrenia suggests that families receiving support may expect the member with schizophrenia to relapse less and be in hospital less. Measuring the impact on admissions and re-admissions for schizophrenia was not deemed appropriate because of the small numbers involved. These data will be monitored once the pilot stage of the work is complete and the family support worker role is rolled out to the rest of the district.

There were 63 referrals to the service, 29 from seven community psychiatric nurses (ranging from one who made nine referrals to single referrals from two), and from voluntary organisations, day hospital and social workers. Fifteen referrals considered outside the project's area were offered a limited service.

Most carers were females or couples caring for an older child (51), with about half being unemployed or retired, and a further quarter housewives. Many carers suffered psychological problems (e.g. stress, anxiety, panic attacks) or practical ones (e.g. inadequate housing, financial difficulties). Emphasis was on practical input, emotional support and information provision.

Later referrals brought in carers of newly diagnosed sufferers whose needs included information about the illness, medication, services and coping with stress and anxiety. These later referrals had more successful outcomes, in terms of sense of control for carers and improved quality of life – especially where the carer was a marital partner with the sufferer having developed symptoms later in life and able to retain better social functioning.

In general, a variety of practical and emotional inputs from the family support worker has led to a range of benefits in terms of service engagement and enhanced quality of life. Examples include:

- an elderly (85-year-old) carer of a 59-year-old son with schizophrenia for 40 years: intensive practical and emotionally supportive counselling has led to improved health and quality of life for the carer (who was treated for depression)
- middle-aged parents of daughter (36 years) with schizophrenia and her son (8 years): involvement with family around medication, illness and with statutory services (e.g. to obtain disability living allowance) led to practical improvements (home renovations), better healthcare (e.g. medication review) and better physical health
- family of daughter (19 years old) suffering from paranoia and threatening suicide: family involvement led to medication review, altering prescribing and referral to

clinical psychologist. Information about medication and services led to involvement of community psychiatric nurse and the family were able to claim disability living allowance. The daughter has returned to college part time and the family have been able to take their first holiday for three years.

As testimony to the success of the project, and to its status locally, the health authority has decided to employ two further family support workers.

THE ERADICATION OF *HELICOBACTER PYLORI* IN THE MANAGEMENT OF DYSPEPSIA

Three projects focused on the eradication of *Helicobacter pylori* (H. *pylori*). Each project had a different approach to the task, with one project being a joint endeavour between a health authority and two NHS trusts (Bradford), one based in an independent applied research unit (Bromley) and one based in a health authority (Walsall).

To set the context for the descriptions of the work in the three projects the following sections answer the questions 'what is the evidence?' and describe how the task of measuring impact was tackled in the three projects. They are followed by notes about each project.

What was the evidence base for the work?

Dyspepsia accounts for a significant proportion of GP workload, prescribing costs and referral to hospitals for diagnostic tests and treatment. It has been estimated that around one in five patients who have dyspepsia also have peptic ulceration. The role of H. *pylori* in the relapse of peptic ulceration is well established as is the marked reduction in relapse that is achieved with eradication of the infection.

The synthesised results from randomised controlled trials of H. *pylori* eradication therapy (triple therapy plus acid-suppressing medicine or amoxycillin plus omeprazole) show that H. *pylori* eradication is highly efficient when using eradication therapy. Ulcer healing rates at 6–10 weeks are significantly better with eradication therapy compared with the short-term use of acid-suppressing drugs alone, and more ulcers are cured at one year with eradication therapy compared with short-term use of acid-suppressing medicine.

Effectiveness Matters, published in 1995, argued that '*Clinicians and managers should ensure that a clear policy and treatment protocols are developed in primary and secondary care for the investigation, diagnosis and treatment of patients with suspected peptic ulcer disease and* H. pylori'

H. pylori *eradication: key references*

- The University of York NHS Centre for Reviews and Dissemination. Helicobacter and peptic ulcer. Effectiveness Matters September 1995; vol 1, issue 2
- Briggs *et al*. Cost effectiveness of screening for and eradication of Helicobacter pylori in the management of dyspeptic patients under 45 years of age. BMJ 1996; 312: 1321–5.

- Hallissey *et al.* Early detection of gastric cancer. BMJ 1990; 301:513–5
- Misiewicz JS *et al.* One week low dose triple therapy for eradication of H. pylori: A large multicentre randomised trial. Gut, 1996; 38 suppl.1.
- Moore A. Helicobacter pylori and peptic ulcer. A systematic review of effectiveness and an overview of the economic benefits of implementing what is known to be effective. 1995; Oxford: Health Technology Evaluation Association.
- Veldhuyzen van Zanten SJO, Sherman PM. Helicobacter pylori infection as a cause of gastritis, duodenal ulcer, gastric cancer and non-ulcer dyspepsia: a systematic overview. Can Med Assoc J 1994; 150:177–185.

What changed?

The three projects focused mainly on changing primary care practice in the management of patients with dyspepsia. Where indicated, patients with proven peptic ulcer disease were tested for the presence of *H. pylori*; if positive, the chosen eradication regime was used to eradicate the infection. Because the drugs used in the eradication 'cocktail' are also used extensively for non-*H.-pylori*-related illness, the use of dose-specific clarithromycin and metronidazole was monitored. The dose-specific data were found to be a good marker for triple therapy prescribing. The impact of eradication on acid-suppressing therapies such as H2 antagonists and proton pump inhibitors was also studied. Because these drugs are used for other non-*H.-pylori*-related illness, no appreciable reduction in the levels of prescribing for these drugs was likely. The impact is also weakened by the significant proportion of patients presenting with so-called 'dual disease', those who have proven ulcer disease associated with *H. pylori* and who also suffer from reflux.

Serology testing and appropriateness of referral were monitored to provide an indication of the take-up of guidelines by general practitioners and also to determine changes in GP understanding of referral protocol.

The measures chosen to measure the impact of the *H. pylori* eradication projects were:

- *Prescribing data*   *Clarithromycin (250mg X 14)**
                                           Metronidazole (400mg X 14) *
                                           H2 antagonists*
                                           Proton pump inhibitors*
- *Diagnostic testing*   *Serology referrals*
- *Referral activity*   *Appropriateness of referral*

Notes about the changes achieved in each of the three projects follow in the project descriptions below.

Reference: PACT data _____

Bashford NR, Norwood J, Chapman SR. Why are patients prescribed proton pump inhibitors? Retrospective analysis of link between morbidity and prescribing in the General Practice Research Database. BMJ 1998; 317:452–456.

Bradford

Why was the project set up?

Discussions at a workshop in July 1995 provided the background to the development of an action plan to tackle clinical and cost-effectiveness in the NHS in Bradford. The action plan proposed a number of clinical topics as priorities for attention and as exemplars for future work on implementing change in clinical practice. Strong evidence for interventions and the probability of success were important factors in selecting the clinical topics. Dyspepsia was one of the topics proposed and one on which the MAAG had already undertaken a primary care audit.

What happened?

Patients with proven duodenal ulcers who were receiving long-term H2 antagonists were chosen as the first stage of this project. Where appropriate, they would be offered eradication therapy for *H. pylori*. The first task for the Bradford project was therefore to produce guidelines to facilitate the identification of those patients whose treatment merited review. The guidelines would also address the broader issue of the management of dyspepsia and the assessment and treatment of new patients.

The project team were aware from the very beginning of the hostile attitudes of some local clinicians towards guidelines. To counter this attitude the development process was made as open as possible and undertaken by clinicians from primary and secondary care working together. Visits to practices by local gastroenterologists and established educational networks were used to promote consistent messages about the work. Local gastroenterologists contributed also to a series of local workshops which were arranged for other local staff, including community pharmacists. *While time-consuming, these discussions strengthened the relationships and partnerships between consultants and GPs – they could now put a name to a face!*

Reviews of evidence produced by national bodies were used as the starting point for the work – rather than seeking to replicate the review process locally. This approach ensured clarity about those elements of the local guidelines which were evidence-based (with evidence displayed and graded to reflect its strengths) and those elements which were consensus-based. *GPs welcomed evidence-based guidelines as preferable to those based largely on clinical opinion. As the work was taken forward, careful thought was given to the presentation of the guidelines to support prescribing decisions.* For example, prompts were built into a computer template which supported the guidelines and new referral forms. These elements formed a single, integrated package.

A group of patients were invited to help with the development of an information leaflet for patients. This task proved to be more difficult than envisaged and with hindsight more time should have been set aside for it: it should have been started earlier. More time should also have been devoted to the needs of Asian patients.

A baseline of current practice against which the impact of the project could be measured was established through audits in primary and secondary care.

After the guidelines and aims of the project had been discussed with practices, the practices were asked to review the treatment of patients receiving long-term H2 antagonists on repeat prescriptions. Audits show that over 1300 patients with peptic ulcer disease were identified and, following re-audit (of 705 patient records), 49 per cent were given eradication therapy.

Management of the project was shared in a core team between the project leader – a consultant in epidemiology and public health based in one of the local NHS trusts – and the project manager – the MAAG manager based at the health authority. *This core team linked the research skills of the project leader with the knowledge of local networks and practices of the project manager and proved invaluable.* There were, however, pros and cons associated with employing the MAAG manager as the project manager. On the positive side, the links and relationships already established provided a sound foundation for the work – the negative was a lack of 'protected time' and thus problems in managing competing workloads.

The core team was supported by a wider project group which involved recognised local clinical leaders from primary and secondary care. *This group deliberately set aside time 'for reflection' so that they could identify, systematically, what they had learned about implementing change – and to review successes and failures. This process proved to be valuable in ensuring that progress was maintained.* For example, it identified one aspect of the work which might have been tackled differently: the handling of the service implications of the project (the need for additional breath tests). *Earlier involvement of service planning managers might have allowed prompter resolution. Making sure that services could cope with the practice changes proved essential.*

A checklist to support further work on guidelines has been a by-product of the work, which will be of real value as plans are rolled forward to build on what has been learned so far. A series of 'PACE educational events' is already planned for primary care groups – to complement the regular GP education programme. These sessions will be 'problem-based' and involve evidence-based guidelines, audit and education. More educational visits to practices by hospital consultants are also planned. Eleven clinical topics will be tackled in the next two years: these include several tackled by other PACE projects, such as back pain and the management of stable angina, as well as others, such as depression, diabetes and epilepsy.

What changed?

Figures 3.14–3.17 provide information related to the agreed measures available in November 1998.

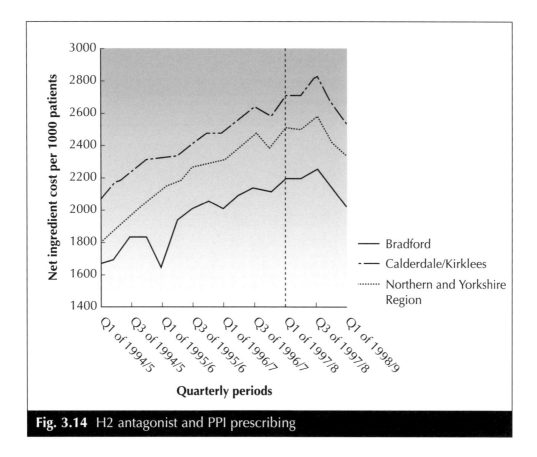

Fig. 3.14 H2 antagonist and PPI prescribing

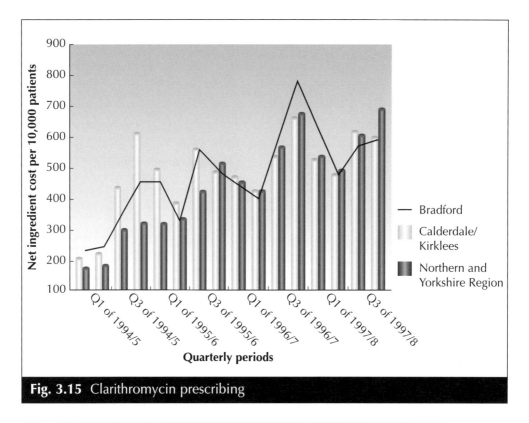

Fig. 3.15 Clarithromycin prescribing

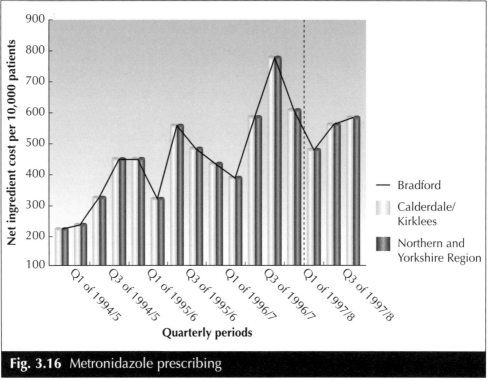

Fig. 3.16 Metronidazole prescribing

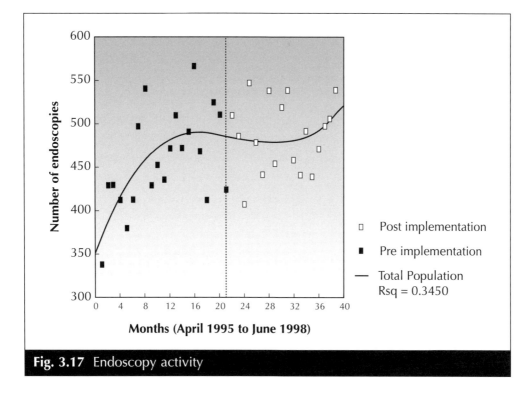

Fig. 3.17 Endoscopy activity

Bromley

Why was the project set up?

During 1995 the health authority and hospital trust established an applied research unit to support the development of evidence-based practice across primary and secondary care. The treatment of peptic ulcers was chosen for attention because it was of major interest to local clinicians, the evidence for change was clear, and there was a high level of expenditure on anti-ulcer drugs. The need for collaborative work between primary and secondary care to implement change made it a practical topic of choice for work by the unit.

What happened?

From the start, the project took a 'hands-on' approach to supporting implementation across primary and secondary care. *The early focus was on six 'pilot' general practices,* chosen as broadly representative in terms of practice population and prescribing patterns.

Attention to detail was important. The team were clear about what they wanted from participants with each head partner receiving a specific contract and payment. The invitation to practices was signed by three key local opinion leaders, the director of public health, the MAAG chair and the senior local gastroenterologist. Project team members gave careful thought to how they presented themselves to practices and about their potential impact as stereotypical manager or commissioner! *The serious point is that establishing credibility is a key to achieving trust and commitment to change.* The joint status of the project between health authority and trust was also important.

Reflecting the need to involve all stakeholders, *the steering group included major decision-makers*, such as consultants, managers, GPs and pharmacists, though *the omission of practice nurses was later considered a mistake*. Meetings were informal and intended as a discussion forum, allowing time for reflection, as well as for decision-making.

As the work with practices was being planned, guidelines needed to be developed – but the team were keen to build on what had been done elsewhere. *They wanted to avoid being tempted into rigorous literature searching and appraisal of the topic in general.* Instead, by engaging practices using a series of case scenarios, the team highlighted divergent current practice and generated debate that led to a more focused search for evidence in areas of disagreement.

Two main strands of work supported the work with practices. First, small group sessions using practical examples enabled lead GPs to explore the benefits of change for practices and patients. Second, the project team helped practices to identify patients whose current treatment needed review. The advantages of participation to general practice in terms of time, money and reduced future consultations were a major selling point. For secondary care clinicians and managers the motivations differed, these stakeholders were particularly sensitive to how change might affect the demand for services.

The advantages of piloting the project included being able to demonstrate a proven and practicable system for change, providing an indication of the resources required to implement the programme and establishing through experience the case for additional resources necessary for Hp testing. *The team recognised that the pilot meant changing the project timetable to allow lessons from the pilot to influence wider implementation.*

The launch of the district-wide 'implementation programme' at a PGEA-accredited evening highlighted that this was not just a set of guidelines, but an 'implementation package'. The package included support for practices to carry out the work by offering the services of a community pharmacist, payment for an in-house practice nurse or practice manager, or a drug-company-sponsored nurse. The variety of options recognises the diversity of GP practices.

The constant challenges were the practicalities of the work rather than philosophy. Applying critical appraisal skills, for example, was less of a problem than how to provide adequate resources, establish appropriate services to support the change, or secure support from local opinion leaders. Other challenges included how to balance work on developing patient information with resources for other activities. *Bearing all these factors in mind, the team concluded that a credible implementation programme in primary care would take at least one year.*

The team concluded that designing a system for change is not difficult. Even getting stakeholders to agree to it may not be that hard. The major headache is finding the resources and practical support to implement change. For example, who will do the actual work of analysing the practice computer or reviewing patients' notes? Who will review medication, discuss changes with patients, and alter long-term prescribing? Many implementation projects seek to motivate general practice staff to do the work themselves, but the lesson from this project is that without support, change simply would not happen.

Finally, the best way of sustaining change is to recognise that *the main investment is the people involved*, ranging from project team members and the steering group, to multi-professional 'implementers'. Recognising the personal motivation of these key people and enabling them to use their participation to develop new skills, complete courses of study and make their current work more varied are important. The experience and expertise of these people will be key to the success of future quality initiatives.

What changed?

The levels of Clarithromycin and Metronidazole prescribing, indicated by net ingredient costs for pilot and non-pilot practices, suggest a rise in the use of recommended eradication regimens during the implementation period. At the same time there was a steady reduction in general expenditure on anti-ulcer medication. More specifically, the monitoring of *H. pylori* serology tests illustrates the rise and fall in testing in the pilot practices as appropriate patients are identified and put through the programme. Non-pilot practices show the general rise in *H. pylori* tests as local and national information impacts on general behaviour.

Figures 3.18–3.21 provide information related to the agreed measures available in November 1998.

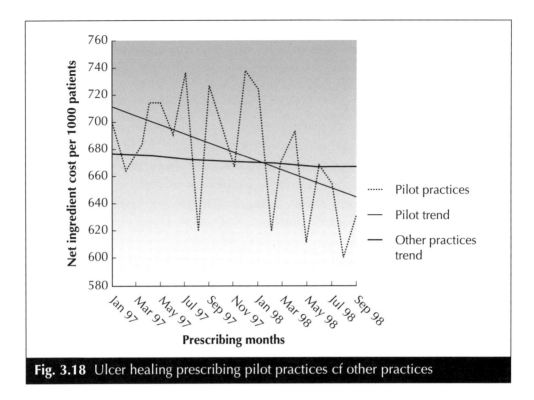

Fig. 3.18 Ulcer healing prescribing pilot practices cf other practices

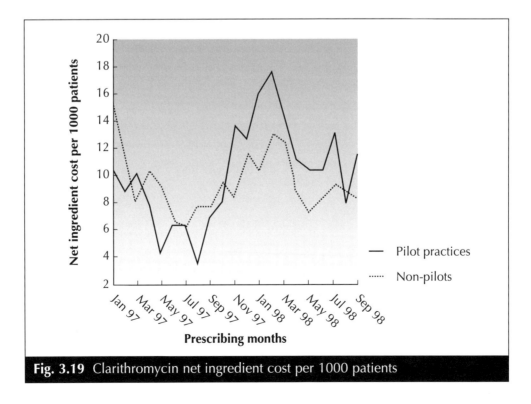

Fig. 3.19 Clarithromycin net ingredient cost per 1000 patients

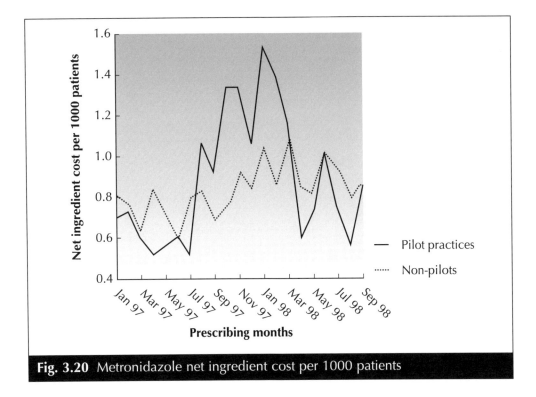

Fig. 3.20 Metronidazole net ingredient cost per 1000 patients

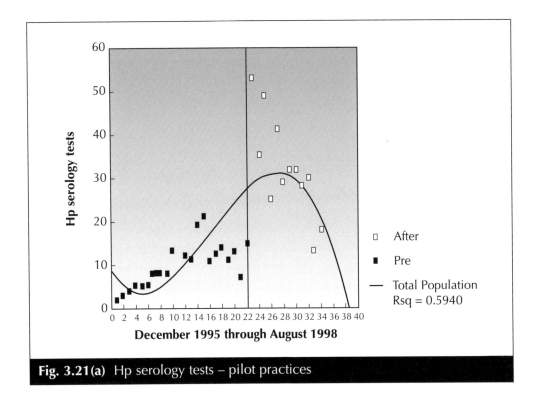

Fig. 3.21(a) Hp serology tests – pilot practices

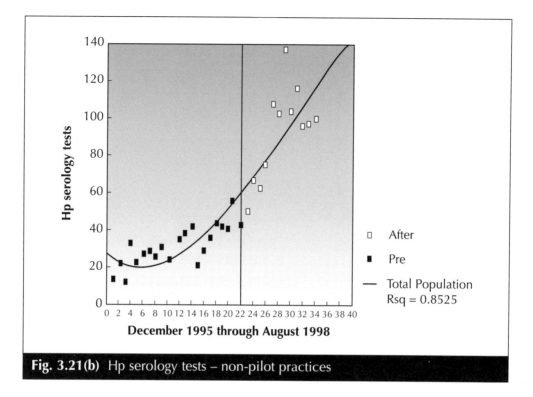

Fig. 3.21(b) Hp serology tests – non-pilot practices

Walsall

Why was the project set up?

In 1995, consultation about the management of upper gastrointestinal disease, between local GPs, the gastroenterologist, the pharmaceutical adviser and a public health consultant, had already taken place. However, this initiative had been put on hold following staff changes. The launch of the PACE programme provided an opportunity to relaunch the work with a specific focus on H. *pylori* eradication in existing patients with peptic ulcer disease.

What happened?

Local discussions had shown that most GPs were antagonistic to the notion of 'guidance' or 'guidelines', preferring the term 'clinical management pathway'. To reflect this concern, suitable material was developed in partnership with gastroenterologists, GP educators, audit groups and Keele University. This material focused on the management of upper gastrointestinal disease across primary and secondary care. To seek consensus, the GPs developing the clinical management pathways included members of the local medical committee and the MAAG. However, in spite of this, neither group considered that they had been adequately consulted. A 'dyspepsia pack', which included laminated copies of the clinical management pathway, was also developed.

In parallel to the work on the *clinical management pathway*, plans were made for an *educational programme*, procedures were set up for *collecting and analysing data* and for developing *monitoring systems*. In addition, plans were made for *identifying patients* in individual primary care practices whose treatment may require review to accord with the pathway and to develop *information for patients*.

The *educational* strand of the work built on a team of pharmacist facilitators from the University of Keele (IMPACT) to promote and explain the clinical pathway to individual GPs and practices. This was an important and successful component of the programme. Educational events included postgraduate meetings, dissemination via MAAG, audit groups and consultant gastroenterologist, and meetings for GPs. A dedicated specialist nurse in gastrointestinal disease who contributed to clinical and educational work with practice nurses was another of the programme's successes. The project team recognised a dilemma with 'educational' events. Although research indicates that formal presentations (lectures), for example, by a consultant to GPs, have limited effectiveness in changing clinical behaviour, they seem to be popular with and emblematic for GPs.

Collecting *baseline data*, particularly in secondary care, proved to be a particular stumbling block that threatened to undermine the project. The system for open-access endoscopies, which was designed to provide reports to GPs, was efficient for administrative purposes only. It did not create meaningful, aggregated information and was not integrated with other systems. Data were held as free-text. To add insult to injury, the person who designed the system and was working on an analysis package left for a new job! The trust was reluctant to continue to develop a stand-alone system and it was difficult to gain consensus from clinicians undertaking endoscopies on a data collection method. These problems led to delays in receiving data and the necessity to rely on crude measures for referrals. Secondary care data collection seemed to be a 'black hole'.

In primary care, it had been planned that the specialist nurse in gastrointestinal disease would advise on patients with hiatus hernia and reflux but the numbers involved meant that the detailed review was restricted to those patients suitable for *H. pylori* eradication. Even so, the resources for such activities should not be underestimated. Although only three practices had completed case-finding by July 1997, these generated enough work to occupy the specialist nurse for over a year.

Work on a patient information booklet drew on results from three patient panels organised by the University of Birmingham and the department of public health. Although this work was delayed, the material was available to support the specialist nurse work in primary care. A major challenge in future will be to ensure that such materials reach the relevant group of patients.

A deliberate *decision was taken not to recruit a project manager to see whether the approach could be incorporated within routine, 'day-to-day' work: 'Possible but difficult' was the verdict.* Managing the work was a continual struggle. The apparently reasonable plan made excessive demands and the inevitable staff changes made matters worse. In hindsight, the project would have benefited from dedicated 'time': ideally from someone with clinical, project management and administrative expertise.

Local medico-political issues strongly inhibited the project's progress, with a degree of un-cooperation arising from some pre-existing tensions between some groups. The formation of working groups on specific aspects of the project also proved difficult and organising meetings was hampered by clinical and other managerial commitments.

The day-to-day work on the project proceeded in an informal, *ad hoc* way and tended to be reactive. Nevertheless, subsequent discussions locally on quality initiatives, such as clinical governance, have begun to refer to the need to draw lessons from PACE. However, any future work will have to tackle the ambivalence of GPs to 'top-down' priority setting and the continued difficulties in co-ordinating work across the primary-secondary care interface. It will also have to draw on the persistence and enthusiasm of dedicated (clinical and managerial) individuals and find ways to secure *and* retain senior level support.

What changed?

Figures 3.22–3.25 provide information related to the agreed measures available in November 1998.

Dyspepsia disease management programme direct access endoscopy referrals

GP Priority/ Guidance priority	Apr 96 to Sep 96	Oct 96 to Mar 97	Apr 97 to Sep 97	Oct 97 to Mar 98
Routine/Routine	6.00	29.00	38.00	37.00
Soon/Routine	1.00	23.00	10.00	5.00
Soon/Soon	1.00	11.00	12.00	11.00
Urgent/Routine	1.00	8.00	4.00	8.00
Urgent/Urgent	6.00	17.00	25.00	32.00

Fig. 3.22 Direct access endoscopy referrals – Audit of priority: April 1996–March 1998

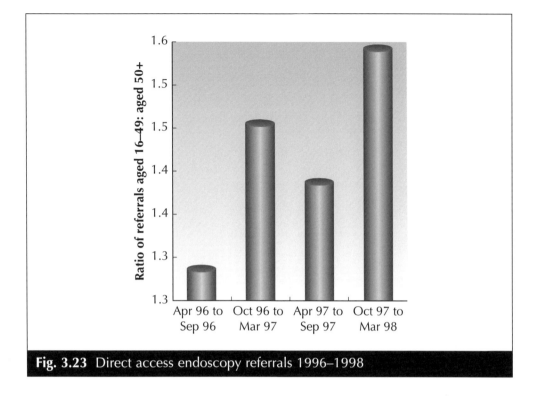

Fig. 3.23 Direct access endoscopy referrals 1996–1998

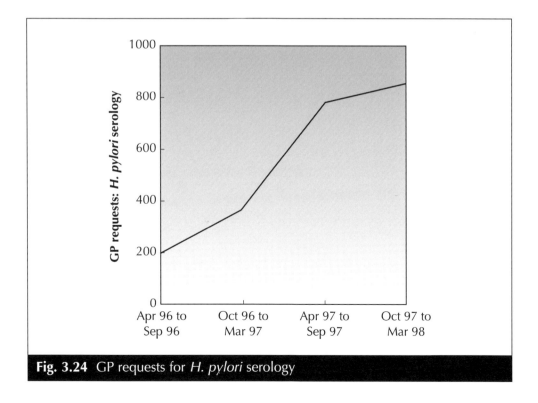

Fig. 3.24 GP requests for *H. pylori* serology

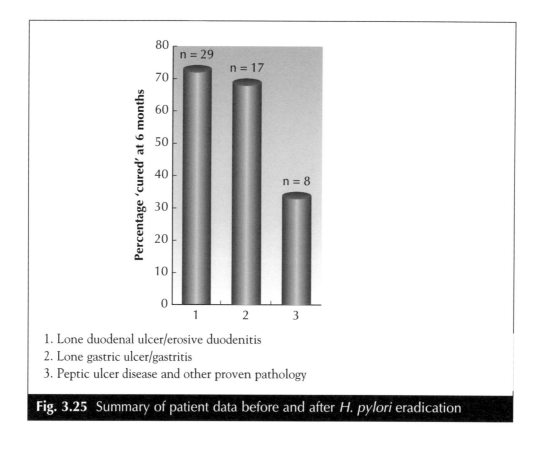

1. Lone duodenal ulcer/erosive duodenitis
2. Lone gastric ulcer/gastritis
3. Peptic ulcer disease and other proven pathology

Fig. 3.25 Summary of patient data before and after *H. pylori* eradication

THE MANAGEMENT OF CONTINENCE

Two projects in the programme were concerned with the management of continence: one was focused on the management of continence in women under 65 (Dudley, whereas the other project was designed to improve district-wide continence services (Wigan and Bolton).

To set the context for these two projects, the following paragraphs answer the question 'What was the evidence base for the work?'

What was the evidence base for the work?

Urinary incontinence is a very common problem, particularly in women. Surveys have shown that up to one in four women suffer from some degree of urinary incontinence. Despite the distressing nature of the problem, many sufferers do not seek medical advice, either because of embarrassment or because they do not realise that effective treatments are available. There is increasing evidence that health gains can be achieved by improving continence services by more accurate diagnosis and appropriate management.

Estimates from other countries on expenditure on continence suggest that incontinence costs 2 per cent of the health budget. Effective treatment, particularly for stress incontinence in women, is usually cheap and simple and prevents the need for lifelong use of expensive incontinence pads. The implementation of research findings should ensure cost savings or at least improved cost-effectiveness.

The management of continence: key references

- Royal College of Physicians. Incontinence: causes, management and provision of services. Report of a working party. London. 1995.
- Agency of Health Care Policy and Research. Urinary incontinence in adults: clinical practice guideline. AHCPR. US Department of Health and Human Services. Rockville, USA. 1992.

Dudley

Why was the project set up?

The management of continence was initially raised at a GP forum in Dudley in 1995 as a major issue of concern. There was recognition of a large unmet need in terms of incontinence prevention and management. These concerns led to the formation of a local working party to explore the issue in more detail. Those discussions in turn led to the development of a PACE project proposal: to focus on urinary incontinence. In particular, to alleviate the distress suffered from this condition by women under 65 years, *deemed to have the largest unmet need with major potential for improvements* with respect to prevention or early treatment.

What happened?

Three streams of activity were created to drive the project forward and establish a strategic approach to the promotion of continence and the management of incontinence. These were focused on raising awareness about the issue, improving the understanding of preventive measures and making treatment more accessible.

Underpinning the project was a *training programme that included educational seminars and the circulation of a continence products directory.* This aimed to ensure nurses could screen women for symptoms of urinary incontinence and manage simple stress incontinence themselves or refer to the continence advisory service. A pre-existing multi-disciplinary continence working party guided the activity with the main work undertaken by the project manager and the local continence adviser. It was decided to adopt *broad objectives for the project to allow flexibility* and this approach proved to be wise because two major issues arose almost straightaway.

First, it was assumed that it would be easy to find practices to pilot the work. In fact, that was the hardest part! Second, to recognise that the project entailed *asking staff not just to change ways of work, but to take on an additional workload*, at least in the short term. Practice nurses did not want to get involved without knowing exactly what was expected of them. The team had to produce, earlier than they had planned, a draft training pack to demonstrate the work involved. *Primary care staff were also reluctant to get involved in data collection*, until collection sheets were tailored to suit them and doubled up as a patient record.

But it was not all bad news. The project staff's *credibility built on their 'knowing the patch', understanding local organisations, knowing key personnel and making the most of existing networks. Offering training sessions at practice premises proved to be a good way of getting practices involved. Enthusiasm for the project became infectious with demonstrated tangible benefits to patients and to staff.* The arrangements for the advisory group meetings ensured that the lessons from the work were identified and shared widely, for example in the distribution of reports and through meetings with senior staff. *Later, as the project moved on, staff from pilot sites became advocates of the work and persuaded colleagues in other practices to join in.*

The team put a lot of energy into public awareness strategies: the topic left many local clinicians uninterested. The stigma attached to the problem also inhibited women coming forward for care. Awareness-raising events – promoting the use of pelvic floor exercises – complemented the development of patient information leaflets. Dissemination had to be tackled imaginatively, for example, by using toilet stickers. Practical considerations proved to be more difficult to resolve than the content of the leaflets. Uncertainty about the management of the continence advisory service led to questions about the use of logos and telephone numbers on posters and leaflets.

Patients' views also helped to shape the development of the service: user and patient focus groups confirmed that women preferred to discuss continence problems with a woman and a nurse. Many didn't want medical interference.

The constant challenge was to keep the message simple, and communicate it sensitively – particular care was needed with humour, and cultural and ethnic issues. Using a local health authority newspaper proved useful in getting messages across rather than persuading the local media to cover the project's story. A real concern was that a successful campaign might overwhelm the continence service: it might become an expensive continence-pad provider.

Some other challenges might have been avoided – others were, perhaps, inevitable, such as staff and organisational changes. It became clear that more attention should have been paid to practice nurses who actually do the work rather than to GPs who organise it. The project was also dogged by bad luck in terms of staff shortages and sickness. Existing continence advisory staff were unable to dedicate the time required and attempts to arrange a secondment failed. A new continence adviser was appointed to co-ordinate the work but she had to act up when the senior continence adviser went on long-term sick leave.

Despite the many challenges, the team held their focus and kept the project moving forward. They even identified and tackled additional issues in response to local needs, for example to create a self-help leaflet for men and to work with a local residential home. Time was *the* real problem – without protected time, things would have been harder and perhaps impossible. Everything took longer and involved more than anticipated. Without the consistent input from the project manager, continence advisers and health promotion advisers, the project would have collapsed. The continence promotion model is now incorporated into a service specification with staff continuity a vital element to success and sustainability. The continence adviser is now a permanent member of staff and educational activity is seen as an ongoing process.

What changed?

Because of the nature of the topic it was difficult to identify routine data for measurement purposes. Clinical audits needed to be undertaken to assess implementation of the guidelines and of the various educational interventions. In addition to these audit activities, the following indicators were also monitored.

- Costs   *Age-specific pad expenditure*
                            Expenditure on aids and appliances
- Referral activity   *Age-specific referrals for stress incontinence*
                            (numbers and appropriateness)

Figures 3.26–3.27 provide the information available in November 1998 for these measures.

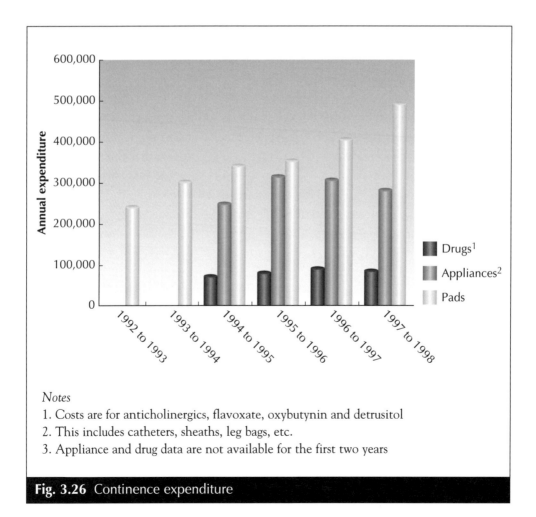

Notes
1. Costs are for anticholinergics, flavoxate, oxybutynin and detrusitol
2. This includes catheters, sheaths, leg bags, etc.
3. Appliance and drug data are not available for the first two years

Fig. 3.26 Continence expenditure

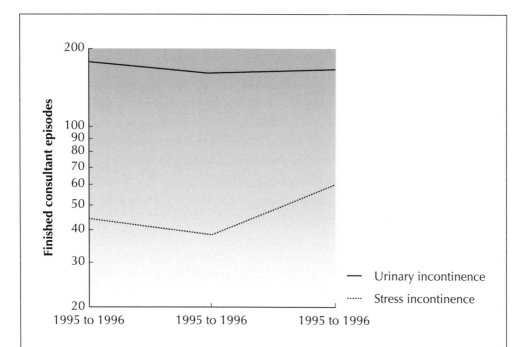

Notes

Number of episodes for urinary incontinence (primary diagnosis) has remained stable.
Number of episodes associated with a procedure for stress incontinence is small and has
remained stable.

Perineometer readings

	Assessment	*1st follow-up (6 weeks)*
Median distress score 6 (0–10)	4 (0–10)	p=0.0019
Perineometer reading 4 (0–8) (range)	6 (0–10)	p<0.0001

Fig. 3.27 Hospital activity for incontinence

Wigan and Bolton

Why was the project set up?

A number of local studies had demonstrated the need for action to improve continence services, for example a study in Wigan in 1995 had demonstrated the high prevalence of incontinence in nursing and residential homes. Meanwhile, in Bolton, long waiting lists for incontinence pads were causing concern and had been criticised by the community health council and local media. Clinical audits also indicated deficiencies in the assessment of people who were receiving incontinence pads. This information led the health authority to make a commitment to improve local services.

What happened?

The studies and concerns which had prompted the need for action across the district had also identified the differences in services in the two main towns – Wigan and Bolton. The absence of a well-established continence service and the high prevalence shown in the survey in nursing and residential homes encouraged initial attention to be focused on Wigan. Services and practice in Bolton were the second stage of the project.

The overall approach endorsed by the health authority was to use the implementation of research evidence as a means to improve the continence service. A secondary aim was to develop a local framework for the implementation of evidence-based practice. *The principle running through the project was that a fundamental change in the philosophy of continence services was required, away from the provision of materials to an emphasis on assessment and treatment.*

Two tasks were tackled in parallel in each stage of the project. First, *the work was planned so that services would be in place prior to any increase in demand.* A service specification was agreed to reflect the main objectives of the project. Subsequently, resources have been allocated to back up these specifications.

Second, a local education programme was organised. A range of materials was developed to support this programme, including evidence-based guidelines, assessment forms and treatment plans and a patient information booklet.

The guidelines were developed by a multi-disciplinary group and cover management in primary care and the reasons for referral to secondary care. The guidelines led to a redesign of the documentation used by community nurses for assessing continence – which had been predominantly used to obtain continence pads. The new documentation has since been used in Bolton Hospital as the basis for a new nursing-care plan. This integrates the hospital and community assessment and has improved communications about referral. In Wigan the option of using the new assessment forms as a referral letter to secondary care has been less successful.

Gaining the support of GPs was tackled by offering GP evening meetings as part of the postgraduate education programmes. Training was also offered to community and practice nurses – with the consultant urologist leading the sessions in Bolton. Community pharmacists were involved because patients often see them as the first source of advice. *Consistency of advice to patients was seen as essential.* All these activities have raised awareness of the issues of clinical effectiveness – as well as questions about continence across the district.

Members of the multi-disciplinary steering group were enthusiastic volunteers. The two key members were the project leader – a consultant in public health medicine, and the project manager – a clinical nurse specialist in gynaecology. The project leader was a local GP and (at the time of the project) medical director of Community Healthcare Bolton. The project manager was a credible source of clinical expertise who later became a clinical nurse specialist in continence and manager of the continence advisory service. Interestingly, these *two people worked in different 'rival' trusts and steps had to be taken to ensure that this situation did not get in the way of progress.* Explicit messages were given to stress the wider aims of the project work, i.e. to promote a collaborative approach to evidence-based practice. *In fact, far from being a problem, the project seems to have benefited from this innovative style of shared leadership.*

Continence did not arouse debate to the extent of other clinical effectiveness topics. Ironically, this lack of controversy combined with acceptance of the evidence resulted in general acceptance of the guidelines. The continence services have also benefited from strong senior management support within the trusts and the commitment of key consultant gynaecologists and urologists. This positive environment has raised the profile of the problem of continence.

Getting messages about the project to other parts of local organisations was achieved through *existing channels*, such as team briefings, practice nurse meetings, GP newsletter and trust professional forum. *Reports were also published in the local press and the project was promoted at a sponsored 'pelvic floorathon'.* Experience later showed that the steering group *might have benefited from involvement by incontinence sufferers as well as representation from the community health council.*

Despite the success of the project, there are still challenges to be faced. Not all consultants are following the guidelines, although the guidelines are now accepted in all NHS trusts and are part of routine record-keeping. The service specification for continence services in Wigan and Bolton should ensure that changes in the service are maintained and training for continence assessment has been made mandatory for community nurses in Community Health Care Bolton. Plans are also in hand to ensure that the lessons learned are used as other work on clinical topics is taken forward locally.

What changed?

The project commenced in Wigan in May 1996 (guidelines were launched in January 1997) and in Bolton in May 1997 (guidelines were launched in February 1998). Because of the nature of the topic, it was difficult to identify routine data for measurement purposes. Clinical audits needed to be specifically undertaken to assess implementation of the guidelines and of the various educational interventions. In addition to these audit activities, the following indicators were also monitored.

- *Prescribing data*   *Anticholinergics*
- *Prevalence targets*   *Wigan: 10 per cent reduction in prevalence of urinary incontinence in nursing and residential homes*
                              Bolton: 10 per cent reduction in the number of people requiring continence materials
- *Assessment targets*   *Wigan and Bolton: 95 per cent assessment of patients receiving continence materials*
- *Materials/costs*   *Pads*
- *Referral activity*   *Numbers and appropriateness*
                              Urodynamics

Figure 3.28 and the following paragraphs provide information related to the agreed measures available in November 1998.

Reduction in the prevalence of incontinence in nursing and residential homes

Visits by the continence advisory service to 24 (out of 40) residential homes by March 1998, confirmed a recorded prevalence of 14 per cent (range 4–44 per cent): 21 per cent of the total residents in these homes (total 625) were assessed.

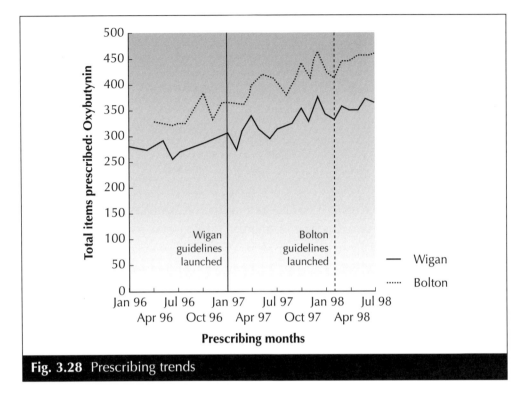

Fig. 3.28 Prescribing trends

Reduction in the number of people requiring continence materials

Wigan	Receiving supplies	Waiting list
September 1996	2200	0
June 1998	1750	0

Reduction = 20%

Bolton	Receiving supplies	Waiting list
July 1997	603	495
October 1998	576	175

Reduction = 4.5% receiving supplies
Reduction = 65% waiting list

Assessment of patients receiving continence materials

Since the start of the project Wigan and Bolton patients cannot be issued continence materials unless a completed assessment form is received. Routine data collection on all patients known to the continence advisory services is still being established.

Monitoring of the services in Wigan: patients receiving pads

Two audits have been undertaken.

	Survey total	Completed questionnaire	Number with completed assessments	Patients who had MSSU
Initial audit	115 (5%)	91 (79%)	22 (24%)	10 (95%)
Repeat audit		50	24 (50%)	20 (84%)

By the time of the second audit it had become apparent that a number of clients were either terminally ill or suffering from dementia. While it was recognised that these clients should receive assessment to exclude a treatable cause of urinary incontinence (e.g. urinary infection or polypharmacy), the guidelines for management in primary care were not felt to be appropriate.

THE CARE AND TREATMENT OF PATIENTS PREDOMINANTLY IN PRIMARY CARE

Three projects were focused on clinical conditions where the main emphasis is on care and treatment in primary care with support from secondary care. The topics were the management of menorrhagia (Dorset), the management of venous leg ulcers (Royal Berkshire) and the care and treatment of patients with low back pain (Southern Derbyshire).

Dorset

Why was the project set up?

In 1994 Dorset Health Authority made a commitment to improving clinical effectiveness – with initial priority being given to establishing an infrastructure for joint working between clinicians and managers. A clinical effectiveness forum was set up to provide *a forum for discussion and action* across the county. The Forum's work included the identification of potential areas for investment or disinvestment based on evidence of clinical effectiveness. In 1995 'dilatation and curettage' (D&C) was identified as a topic for attention and the proposal for a PACE project grew out of these discussions.

What was the evidence base for the work?

Menorrhagia (excessive regular menstrual blood loss) results in considerable numbers of GP referrals to hospital for further management and accounts for over half of all hysterectomies. Half of all the women who have a hysterectomy for menorrhagia have their uterus removed. In the secondary care setting there are wide variations in the management of patients, leading to inconsistencies in decision-making, duplication of treatment and often unnecessary surgical intervention. In primary care one of the most commonly prescribed drugs, norethisterone, is probably the least effective. The evidence suggests that tranexamic acid and mefenamic acid are among the most effective treatments. These anomalies suggest the need for a structured treatment plan and the development of evidence-based guidelines. Since no management option is superior in all respects, women should be assisted to make informed choices about the various treatment options.

The management of menorrhagia: key references ⸻⸻⸻⸻⸻⸻⸻

- Nuffield Institute for Health, Leeds University & NHS Centre for Reviews and Dissemination, University of York. The management of menorrhagia: What are

effective ways of treating excessive regular menstrual blood loss in primary and
secondary care? Effective Health Care. Aug 1995; No 9.

- Lähteenmäki P *et al.* Open randomised study of use of levonorgestrel releasing intrauterine
  system as alternative to hysterectomy. BMJ 1998; 316:1122–6.
- Bonnar J, Sheppard BL. Treatment of menorrhagia during menstruation: randomised
  controlled trial of ethamsylate, mefenamic acid, and tranexamic acid. BMJ 1996;
  313(7057):579–82, Sept 7.
- Coulter A, Kelland J, Peto V, Rees MC. Treating menorrhagia in primary care.
  An overview of drug trials and a survey of prescribing practice. International Journal
  of Technology Assessment in Health Care 1995; 11(3):456–71

What happened?

This project aimed to improve the diagnosis and management of menorrhagia across
primary and secondary care. There were five strands to the work. First, to develop
evidence-based clinical guidelines on the management of menorrhagia. Second, to
promote understanding and adoption of the guidelines Third, to re-audit practice to
check compliance with the guidelines. Fourth, to work with patients to create
information leaflets. Fifth, to develop one-stop diagnostic clinics in each local acute trust.

The starting point for the work was an assessment of the local approaches to the
treatment of menorrhagia. Problems identified included a wide variety of prescribing
practices in primary care and the fragmented nature of treatment provided within
local hospitals. *This knowledge was used to demonstrate the need for change.* A leaflet
about the project was distributed across the county with copies going to every practice,
to hospital staff in gynaecology departments, to pharmacists and to relevant local
groups and committees. Subsequently, all Dorset GPs were sent a questionnaire to
confirm the assessment of current practice and establish their level of understanding
about the evidence base. *A sample of these GPs was invited to comment on the draft guidelines
which were being developed. The covering letter also offered training on the guidelines but
take-up from this offer was poor.*

Guidelines were developed by a clinical outcomes and audit group with particular
care to ensure that those for secondary care were compatible with those for primary
care. *The absence of published national guidelines meant that a considerable amount of time
was spent researching the literature. External funding made this approach possible – without it,
the team doubted whether it would be possible to adopt a similar approach for other guidelines.*

*A major consideration for the team was to find a practical application for the guidelines since
GPs had a choice of hospital to which they could refer.* There was concern that differing
messages from the separate gynaecology teams could undermine the credibility of the
guidelines. The team responded by developing linked clinical pathways and one-stop

menorrhagia clinics were planned for each (of three) local acute trusts. *Standardised referral forms for GPs and a standardised form for reports to GPs from the hospital were developed to support this approach: it had mixed success.* At one hospital, a weekly menorrhagia clinic was established, run by an associate specialist using existing equipment. At another, it proved difficult because the physical environment was unsuitable and there were problems with a lack of specialist nurses and equipment. At the third, progress was slower because of anxieties that a one-stop clinic would not give women sufficient time to prepare for an invasive procedure: arrangements have now been introduced for a specialist nurse to provide information and advice to patients before the appointment.

A *programme of 'road shows'* was organised to explain the evidence, the guidelines and the one-stop clinics. These accredited practice-based training sessions were led by three local gynaecologists. Unlike the attempts to promote the guidelines, *there was good take-up of practice-based sessions and feedback was positive: GPs were pleased that consultants had taken the trouble to lead these sessions.* This 'marketing' approach came to be seen as the essential area of activity. Borrowing from commercial experience, the lessons learned included the need to focus on clear, concise *messages*, use credible and authoritative *messengers*, reach out to clinicians rather than expecting them to come to you, fit into clinicians' busy schedules and *make learning rewarding, light-hearted and fun.*

The work was promoted as a means of reflecting on new research and providing an opportunity to review current practice. The approach meant recognising that clinicians had not been deliberately mistreating their patients. With different levels of interest across the county, it was essential to ensure that enthusiasts were on board and willing to support their colleagues. Offering practical help, such as simple audit tools, was also beneficial. Engaging key people within local networks was important; for example, GP tutors advised on the approach to disseminating the guidelines within primary care.

Working with patients provided valuable insights into the impact the condition (and mistreatment) has on people. Issues of concern included doctors' attitudes and their willingness (or lack of) to explain treatment options in a clear way. The CHC carried out a survey and conducted focus groups to feed into developing a booklet for women on heavy menstrual bleeding. This booklet was circulated to all GP practices and publicised in the local press. The local guidelines were also translated into lay language and distributed to GP practices and outpatient clinics.

The project benefited from *strong commitment from the consultant gynaecologists and GP members of the project team and those on a wider steering group.* The consultants carried the weight and authority in primary care and local GPs appreciated their active involvement.

What changed?

The work encompassed the diagnosis and medical and surgical management of menorrhagia. As well as identifying a number of indicators to measure change in both settings (GP prescribing and surgical interventions in local hospitals), the project also used audit to establish compliance with the guidelines and resulting outcomes.

The measures for the project were:

- *Prescribing (PACT) data*   *Norethisterone per 1000 women aged 30–49*
  Mefenamic acid per 1000 women aged 30–49
  Tranexamic acid per 1000 women aged 30–49
- *Inpatient/day case activity*   *D&C women aged 30–49*
  Endometrial ablation women aged 30–49
  Hysterectomy women aged 30–49

Figures 3.29–3.31 provide information available in November 1998 for these measures.

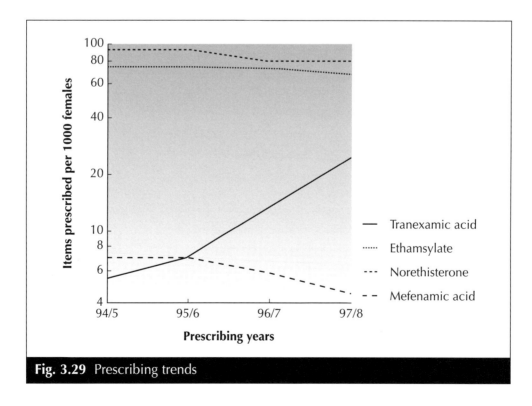

Fig. 3.29 Prescribing trends

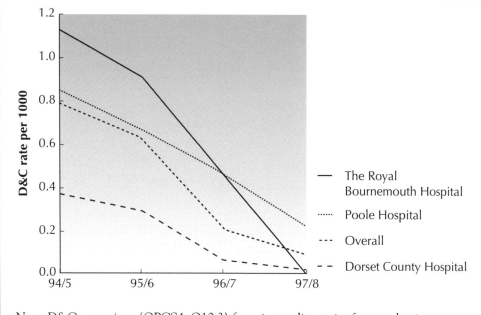

Note: D&C operations (OPCS4, Q10.3) for primary diagnosis of menorrhagia (ICD9 626.2, 627.0; ICD10 N92.0, N92.4). Rate per 1000 women aged 15–55, Dorset Health Authority residents.

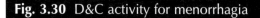

Fig. 3.30 D&C activity for menorrhagia

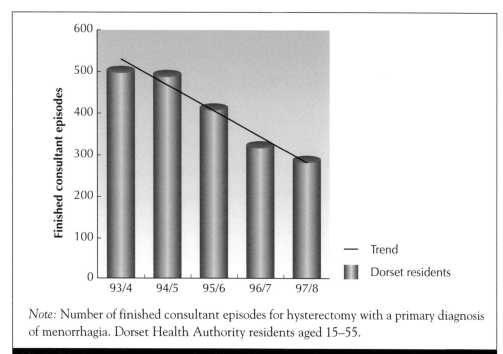

Note: Number of finished consultant episodes for hysterectomy with a primary diagnosis of menorrhagia. Dorset Health Authority residents aged 15–55.

Fig. 3.31 Hysterectomy activity for menorrhagia

Royal Berkshire

Why was the project set up?

A study of a sample of patients with leg ulcers in Berkshire in 1994/95 suggested that for patients who had chronic venous leg ulcer, the average duration of the leg ulcer was ten years, ranging from three months to 40 years. Local practice was judged to be below acceptable standards and action deemed necessary to improve the quality of patient care.

What was the evidence base for the work?

During the past ten years the research carried out into the management of leg ulcers paints a depressing picture of costly and ineffective care provided against a background of uncoordinated and piecemeal services. The evidence also suggests that treatment of the condition is frequently based on inadequate assessment that fails to take into account the ulcer's underlying condition.

Effective treatment outcomes have been achieved where comprehensive assessment of the patients condition precedes a co-ordinated multi-disciplinary approach, such as that provided at a leg ulcer clinic. Treatments which focus on correcting venous hypertension through the use of high compression bandaging increase ulcer healing rates. No clear differences in the effectiveness of different types of high-compression bandaging have been shown.

The management of leg ulcers: key references _____

- Elliot *et al.* 1996; Setting a standard for leg ulcer assessment. Journal of Wound Care. 5:173–5
- Simon *et al.* Community leg ulcer clinics: a comparative study in two health authorities. BMJ, 1996; 312:1648–51
- Cullum *et al.* Compression bandages and stockings in the treatment of venous leg ulcers. (Cochrane review) In: The Cochrane Library, Issue 2. Oxford.

What happened?

Reducing the duration, variation and cost of treating leg ulcers and helping patients to understand the risks about ulceration and be involved in their own treatment were the aims of this project. A multi-disciplinary advisory committee planned the strategic direction and a smaller project team organised the work. From the beginning the plan was to integrate project objectives with those of local professional groups and organisations, to improve co-operation between disciplines, to support team building and to find ways of achieving enduring changes in clinical practice.

Five broad areas were identified for attention, creating an *assessment tool and protocol,* providing *staff education, involving patients, auditing practice* to measure the impact of the work and an *economic analysis.* A communication strategy using existing channels and which shared responsibilities between project team members ensured that all interested parties were kept in touch with progress.

Gaining consensus in the development of an *assessment tool and treatment and referral protocol* was a slow, painstaking process, with more debate about style and design than clinical content. Meetings were impractical, so the project nurse spent many hours discussing drafts with clinicians individually. Parallel action was necessary so that nurses had the education and equipment necessary for accurate assessments. Vascular surgeons now accept direct referrals from nurses and use the assessment form as a basis for their own interventions. The surgeons report a significant improvement in the appropriateness of referrals since the protocol has been used.

Three principles steered the *staff education programme.* First, education was run concurrently and linked with other development work. Second, 'learning by doing' were the watchwords. Third, clinicians got the resources and equipment to do the job. An assessment of educational needs identified three levels of expertise: *specialist* – to assess leg ulcers and make recommendations for management; *practitioner* – to provide knowledge and skills for day-to-day care; and *general* – to promote a positive attitude to leg ulcer management.

Nurses trained to 'specialist' level now act as a local resource. They have access to equipment and educational material and are networked to ensure that their skills and expertise are utilised to the best effect. At 'practitioner' level over 300 nurses have attended sessions: educational exchange visits have enabled nurses from different settings to understand each other's problems. General awareness sessions have been run for all health care professionals. *The educational programme has shown that how diagnosis was established was more important than who made the initial diagnosis.*

Quality of life studies have offered a glimpse into the lives of people suffering from this painful condition and serve as a reminder of patients' low expectations. The team decided that the project needed to be informed by patients' views and secured these through a series of interviews. Liaison with the CHC, the health promotion department and patient groups also helped the preparation of *patient information on leg ulcer care.* These activities helped staff to understand the impact of the condition on patients' lives and led to suggestions for improvements, such as better availability of compression hosiery and better rural transport services. The team has launched a 'healthy legs for life' campaign to build on these experiences.

An audit study was set up to investigate the application of graduated compression bandaging and its effect on the healing of chronic venous leg ulcers within a 12-week period and promote local ownership of the need to change practice. The audit focused on a cohort of 30 patients. In addition, a 'tracking' audit was undertaken to monitor decision-making processes and referrals and treatments for a cohort of patients in acute and community settings. *Both audits demonstrated that graduated compression was clinically effective for leg ulcers.*

The team was continually up against other issues competing for management attention. They kept a careful watch on other developments, particularly relating to resources issues. An *economic evaluation* helped to illustrate the potential financial savings.

The problem of **time** *came through again and again as the project was driven forward – there was never enough of it.* Face-to-face contact, consensus building and protocol development were lengthy processes. Negotiating through organisational structures and communicating with policy committees were delicate tasks, especially where informal practices and covert gatekeeping were common!

The practice development nurses in community and acute trusts plan to carry on working together with a shared programme of leg ulcer events. They are in liaison with the Royal College of Nursing so that recommended practices are kept aligned with national guidelines. Systems will be required to sustain change beyond the life of the project and an infrastructure put in place to support future developments. Based on their experience in the project, practice and community nurses are well equipped to contribute to the development of primary care groups and thus ensure that the delivery of evidence-based care continues to receive attention.

What changed?

Clinical audit was used to investigate the effects on healing leg ulcers within a 12-week period. The effectiveness of the leg ulcer assessment tool and protocol, the impact of staff education and the level of co-operation between various care providers were also assessed. Economic evaluation provided an analysis of current costs within local service providers and provided a basis for assessing the implications for future service developments. The specific measures for this project were:

- *Clinical audit* *Healing outcome audit: Can the application of graduated compression bandaging accelerate the healing of chronic venous leg ulcers within a 12-week period?*

> *Tracking audit: Do patients receive consistent evidence-based management of their ulcer between hospital and community settings?*

* *Economic analysis:*   *Aimed to estimate the hypothesis that total costs of treating leg ulcers will be smaller with the provision of graduated compression, and that this is caused by a reduction in the number of nurse consultations required, in the length of time required in providing care and in the number of nurse visits*

Figures 3.32–3.33 provide information available in November 1998 for these measures.

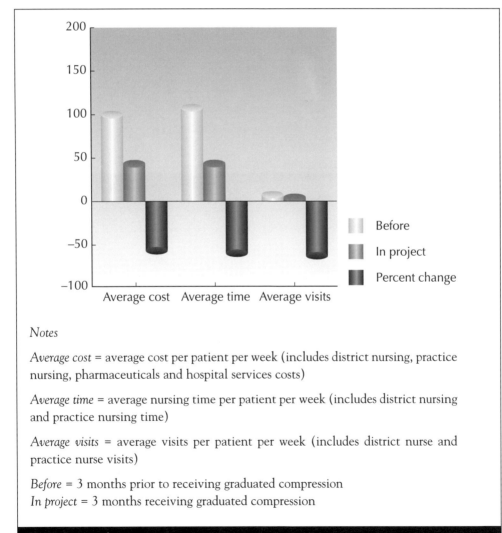

Notes

Average cost = average cost per patient per week (includes district nursing, practice nursing, pharmaceuticals and hospital services costs)

Average time = average nursing time per patient per week (includes district nursing and practice nursing time)

Average visits = average visits per patient per week (includes district nurse and practice nurse visits)

Before = 3 months prior to receiving graduated compression
In project = 3 months receiving graduated compression

Fig. 3.32 Evaluation summary

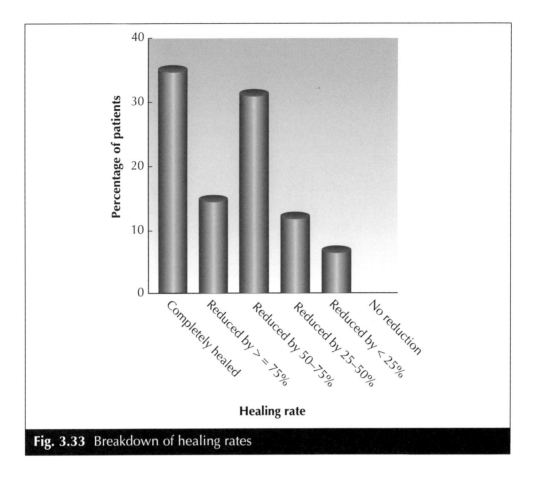

Fig. 3.33 Breakdown of healing rates

Southern Derbyshire

Why was the project set up?

A conference in Derby in early 1995, under the banner 'Shifting Sands', brought together clinicians from across Southern Derbyshire who felt deluged with guidelines and who called for better co-ordinated guideline development. Arising from the discussion at the conference, a clinical development group brought together representatives from primary and secondary care, postgraduate education and clinical audit, health authorities and trusts and patient groups. Low back pain was chosen as one of five clinical issues for attention because of *a groundswell of GP opinion that this was a topic of major concern.*

What was the evidence base for the work?

In the course of a 12-month period, around 7 per cent of adults in the UK consult their GPs with back pain. Of these, around two-thirds are prescribed medication, 10–20 per cent are referred to a hospital doctor or a physiotherapist, osteopath or chiropractor. A significant proportion of people who experience back pain report restrictions in mobility affecting normal activities at work, in the home or in their leisure pursuits. Around 90 per cent of patients with low back pain in primary care will have stopped consulting with symptoms within three months. However, most will still be experiencing low back pain and related disability one year after consultation. Since most 'consulters' continue to experience long-term pain and disability, effective early treatment could reduce the burden of these symptoms and social, economic, and medical impact.

In 1994, the Clinical Standards Advisory Group reported

> *'The importance of primary care management of back pain within the first six weeks cannot be over-emphasised. Once chronic back pain and disability are established, any form of treatment is more difficult and has a much lower chance of success. Early management sets the whole strategy and very largely determines the final outcome. It has a powerful influence on the patient's and family's attitudes and beliefs about the problem and how it should be dealt with'.*

Low back pain: key references _____

- Clinical Standards Advisory Group. Back pain – Report of a CSAG Committee on Back Pain. HMSO. 1994.
- Agency for Health Care Policy and Research. Management guidelines for acute low back pain. AHCPR. 1994
- Macfarlane *et al.* Outcome of low back pain in general practice: a prospective study. BMJ 1998; 316:1356–9
- Ellis R M. Back pain – emphasise early activity and support it with services geared to active management. BMJ 1995; 310:1220.

What happened?

There were two initial strands to the work in this project, first to create a new local 'evidence-based' guideline and second to explore and develop local services to deliver the required level of practice. These tasks were assigned to two task groups whose membership included consultants, GPs, therapists, a chiropractor and an osteopath.

The work on guidelines included standard referral forms to link with the patient record. The guideline also gives advice on management and offers samples of patient information. The strength of the evidence meant easy consensus over the content of the guidelines, but this *early decision to accept the evidence led to an underestimation of the work needed to make a critical assessment of current practice.*

*Ensuring and **demonstrating** that clinical staff were able to provide the level and nature of practice described in the guideline proved to be a more difficult task.* While chiropractors and osteopaths were able to demonstrate the required skills through their professional requirements, this process was less clear for physiotherapists. A programme of professional educational workshops followed. This was accompanied by a booklet containing the guideline and supporting evidence, which was distributed to all local GPs and local services.

The two task groups merged after the guidelines were agreed. *Auditing was recognised as a key activity* in monitoring the process of implementation, with every patient seen by a physiotherapist being subject to audit, while a volunteer group of GPs are auditing their practice. *An independent evaluation of the work was also carried out* by York Health Economics Consortium and the Centre for Health Economics to assess the impact of guidelines and service reconfiguration and to examine the views of stakeholders in relation to the changes. The evaluation also reviewed the extent to which the project had enhanced collaboration locally between primary, secondary care and the health authority.

Communicating the messages about the project has been a feature of the project team's work. An example of this work was a public health occasional paper, which was disseminated widely locally to clinical staff in primary and secondary care. This has been complemented by a concerted effort to help the *public understand the new approach*.

A local '*search conference*' brought together service users, staff from primary and secondary care, the health authority and the voluntary sector to debate the new approach. The aim for the day was to promote an understanding of the issues and a shared vision for future services. Questions addressed at the conference included the nature of current services, whether they matched people's needs and how they could be improved. The conclusions from the day emphasised the need for early accurate diagnosis, early access to appropriate treatment, confusion caused by the myriad approaches to treatment, the need for a holistic approach and accessible specialist co-ordinator to direct patients to treatment.

One intriguing facet of the 'search conference' discussion was *the potential conflict between scientific evidence and patient expectancy.* For example, the guideline emphasises the role of diagnostic triage to eliminate serious pathology and states that there is little value in being specific about the cause of the pain – this was contrary to patients' expectations! Subsequently, a programme of public education was agreed and a survey undertaken to assess knowledge and understanding of the management of back pain. The public education work was backed up with the development of information materials, local media articles and radio features.

Improvements in the local service included the establishment of a rehabilitation service. This became an investment priority for 1998/99. Serious consideration was given to developing a Derby Back Pain Centre (a one-stop shop), but there was concern about the impact of this approach on patients' expectations. This led to the establishment of a 'conceptual' centre as a focus to bring together several strands of clinical practice under an umbrella of agreed standards and referral pathways – rather than as a physical entity.

Ultimately, the project has been dependent on *the commitment and enthusiasm of individuals.* In hindsight, the project team has recognised how easy it is to underestimate the resources needed to change clinical practice and the importance of being more focused on particular changes in practice.

The back pain project is one of five projects in the district. The work will continue to draw on the results of the evaluation by York and the ongoing feedback of the audit results to local clinicians. The change mechanisms are already in place – the standardised referral letter, computerised guidelines and a more systematic approach to practice-based education – and should increasingly bear fruit.

What changed?

The plan was to monitor the appropriateness and number of referrals to physical therapy clinics. Because X-rays for simple back pain are not indicated in routine systems, the plan was to record plane lumber spine activity. Southern Derbyshire also commissioned York Health Economics Consortium to evaluate their work.

The key measures for this project were:

- *Diagnostic testing* *Plane lumber spine X-rays*
- *Referral activity*   *Appropriateness of referral*
         Back pain clinic referrals
         Physiotherapy referrals
- *Inpatient activity*   *Admissions for epidural*

Information was not available at the time that this report went to press to illustrate the scale of change achieved by the project work.

THE CARE OF PATIENTS IN HOSPITAL

Two projects were focused on aspects of the care and treatment of patients while they are in hospital: Chase Farm (the prevention of pressure sores); and Oxfordshire (post-operative pain control).

Chase Farm

Why was the project set up?

In 1995 an *Effectiveness Bulletin*, published by the NHS Centre for Reviews and Dissemination, had reported on the effectiveness of interventions to prevent and treat pressure sores. This publication coincided with a local fact-finding mission, which indicated that local practice showed scope for improvement. These two initiatives stimulated discussions within the trust about the burden of suffering from pressure sores on patients and their carers which in turn led to agreement that action was needed. The plans for the project were aimed at reducing the incidence of hospital-acquired pressure sores and improving the management of existing pressure sores.

What was the evidence base for the work?

Pressure sores are common in hospital and community settings and represent a significant burden of suffering for patients and their carers. For many patients the development of a pressure sore will significantly slow recovery following illness or surgery and for some patients the presence of a sore will lead to complications such as chest infection or urinary infection. For a few the development of a pressure sore may even lead to death. Evidence on the effectiveness and cost-effectiveness of equipment for the prevention and treatment of pressure sores is equivocal.

What evidence there is indicates that an effective approach to the prevention and treatment of pressure sores is likely to encompass some or all of the following elements:

- development of evidence-based guidelines
- use of some form of low pressure foam mattresses or other 'low tech' pressure-relieving method (e.g. 30-degree tilt)
- introduction of pressure sore incidence monitoring and feedback mechanisms (if incidence rates are being used as measures of quality across units, care must be taken to adjust for patients' risk of developing pressure sores)
- routine systems for checking the quality and availability of equipment
- regular audit and feedback.

Pressure sore management: key references _____

- Nuffield Institute for Health, Leeds University, NHS Centre for Reviews and Dissemination – University of York. The prevention and treatment of pressure sores: How effective are pressure relieving interventions and risk assessment for the prevention and treatment of pressure sores. Effective Health Care. October 1995; Vol 2 No 1.
- AHCPR. Clinical practice guideline, pressure sore prevention in adults: prediction and prevention. Silver Spring, Agency for Health Care Policy and Research, U.S. Department of Health and Human Services, 1992.
- Department of Health. Pressure sores: A key quality indicator – A guide for NHS purchasers and providers. London, 1993.
- McSweeney P. Pressure sores: Assessing the cost of pressure sores. Nursing Standard. September 1994; Vol 8 No 52
- Fletcher J *et al*. Mattress replacements: Assessment and evaluation. Journal of Tissue Viability. Calderdale NHS Trust. 1993; Vol 4 No 4

What happened?

The initial tasks to get this project rolling were to complete an audit of pressure care and wound management and to develop local evidence-based guidelines. Related tasks were to improve data collection and review nursing records – and start to plan an educational programme. There were a range of early problems that inhibited rapid progress.

The *absence of a reputable national guideline for pressure sore management proved to be a real 'chasm' that the project team had to cross.* They had to establish a local framework for assembling the evidence and writing the local guideline. The incomplete evidence base was a particular problem with respect to risk assessment and effectiveness of pressure care equipment. The team found that *in the absence of national guidelines it took a significant amount of time and expertise to put together local guidelines.* Understanding the needs of the audience for the guideline material was important and several different formats were needed for the different professional groups: the material included quick reference guides, detailed resource folders and flowcharts.

Some *practical obstacles also had to be overcome, such as limited resources (and desk space!), changes of personnel, and the challenge of fitting in the work with existing work pressures.* Despite all of these problems, the project soon generated enthusiasm locally. *The director of nursing as project leader was essential in influencing and securing the support of key people on the trust board and in the health authority.*

A large multi-professional steering group was set up to oversee the project: membership covered physiotherapy, medicine, pharmacy, business management, surgical appliances, performance management, nursing, audit and education. It was useful to have this large group to oversee the work but working with a large group was difficult: it was often hard to get them together in one room. A smaller (nursing) working party undertook most of the detailed work!

Some months after the project was launched staff changes required a change in project leadership. A nurse with extensive experience of management in a clinical setting – from another NHS trust – was appointed as project co-ordinator. Despite some early reservations about whether someone new to the organisation could co-ordinate this type of work, her clinical background ensured credibility with colleagues, and helped to advance the work quickly. On reflection, the team felt that *the external appointee was particularly successful*. She had time to do the work and was less distracted by other responsibilities – but care was needed to keep broad ownership of the work. The lesson from this is *do not rely too heavily on one person because of the inevitability of staff changes*.

A flexible education programme was introduced to help promote a better understanding of the changes to practice that were needed. These offered nursing staff a mix of classroom and ward-based sessions. The sessions were regularly evaluated to ensure that they were providing the necessary range of information and practical help.

A local wound care group, which included link nurses for each clinical area, helped to disseminate information and review products relating to wound care and pressure sore prevention. Indeed, one of the main ingredients for success of the project was the local *link nurse system* which provides for a pooling of experiences and knowledge and sharing of resources. The Hospital League of Friends proved to be unexpected allies: *think imaginatively about who can be involved to support the work. To help spread the message, the team also 'piggy-backed' on local communication channels*, such as the medical audit group, and reports were included in local newsletters.

The enthusiasm generated by the project was infectious – in one busy acute medical ward (not explicitly part of the PACE initiative) the ward manager and sister decided to address the entire range of issues relating to pressure sores. *This 'zero-tolerance' approach resulted in reports that no patient had developed a pressure sore in six months*.

Despite the best of plans *unforeseen cost implications arose* – such as the need for pressure care equipment. This stressed the need to be *aware of the service and resource consequences of change*. Chase Farm Hospital has since joined a national pressure sore audit and has moved towards an improved pressure sore data analysis system. A new post within the trust of clinical practice facilitator is a manifestation of the commitment to build on the PACE experience and improve the quality of clinical practice in the trust.

What changed?

A number of different ways were adopted to reflect the diversity of the work undertaken during the project and the complexity of the subject itself. An important feature of the work was to establish a system to routinely monitor the incidence of hospital-acquired pressure sores at ward level.

Documentation audits were also carried out at two points through the project. The audits were designed to look at the nursing records relating to the assessment of patients at risk of pressure sore development. The purpose was to identify changes in practice in record keeping as a result of the introduction of the pressure sore policy, the educational programme and the evidence-based resource folders. A year-on-year assessment of dressing cost changes was also carried out.

The specific measures were:

- *Inpatient activity*   *New hospital-acquired pressure sores*
                            Severity of sores
- *Ward-based activity*   *Number of forms actually returned compared with the*
                            number that should have been returned
- *Dressing costs*   *Varidase (1995/6 cf 1996/7) (inpatient hospital prescribing)*

Figure 3.34 shows the fall in hospital-acquired pressure sores between November 1996 and August 1998. Information about other aspects of the evaluation was not available in November 1998.

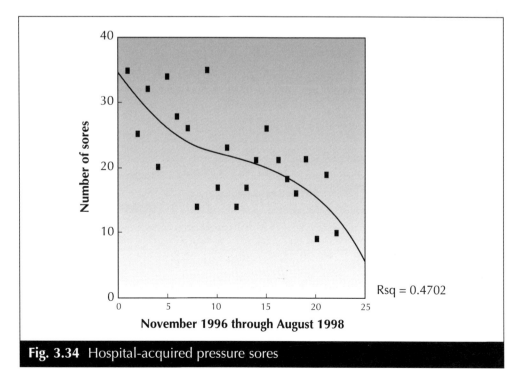

Fig. 3.34 Hospital-acquired pressure sores

Oxfordshire

Why was the project set up?

The results of local studies had persuaded clinicians and managers that there was considerable scope for improvement in the management of post-operative pain in both the John Radcliffe Hospital (part of the Oxford Radcliffe, a university teaching hospital) and the Horton Hospital (a district general hospital). The project aimed to improve the management of post-operative pain in both these hospitals and compare the differences between the two implementation processes. At that time the hospitals were separate trusts, but since the project was set up the two hospitals have become parts of one.

What was the evidence base for the work?

The provision of adequate post-operative analgesia is an essential component of surgical and anaesthetic management of patients who require surgery, and there is much high quality evidence to guide good practice. Despite this, studies have shown that pain management following surgery continues to be inadequate and that patients will still suffer moderate to severe pain. The consequences of untreated pain include an increased incidence of nausea and vomiting, an increased predisposition to respiratory and mobility complications, a stress response and a longer stay in hospital.

The evidence that exists indicates that education and training on pain management and the development of written guidelines on the subject greatly decrease post-operative pain. A multi-centre Department of Health funded audit also confirmed the benefit of simple methods for improving pain control. These include the use of routine pain and sedation scoring and the introduction of an intra-muscular opioid algorithm.

Post operative pain control: key references _____

- Royal College of Surgeons of England, Royal College of Anaesthetists. Report of the working party on pain after surgery. London: Royal College of Surgeons, 1990.
- Agency of Health Care Policy and Research. Acute pain management guideline panel. Acute pain management: operative or medical procedures and trauma. Clinical Practice Guideline. AHCPR. US Department of Health and Human Services. Rockville, USA, 1995.
- Gould TH *et al*. Policy for controlling pain after surgery: effects of sequential changes in management. BMJ, 1992; 305:1187–93.
- Mac Lellan K. A chart audit reviewing the prescription and administration trends of analgesia and the documentation of pain after surgery. Journal of Advanced Nursing 1997; 26:345–350.

What happened?

The introduction of the systematic assessment of pain and sedation, an algorithm for pain management, and use of patient controlled analgesia (PCA) were the activities at the heart of this project. Senior clinicians led project teams at the two hospitals, with the project co-ordinated through a multi-disciplinary steering group led by a public health consultant at the health authority.

At both hospitals, project teams had assembled the evidence before the project work started: the evidence was not controversial. The main challenge was to encourage its use and the two local teams developed and disseminated local guidelines to support this process. Post-operative monitoring forms were amended to include sections on scoring pain and sedation. Information packs were developed covering acute pain management, use of algorithms and PCA. Sequential audits monitored the impact of the work: patient surveys had identified priority areas for improvement.

Education was the main focus for the work at both hospitals. It was a major undertaking with 'education' gaps ranging from fears about patient addiction to worries about well-publicised side-effects. One lead clinician was astonished to learn that surgery finals did not include pharmacology. Nurse seminars were held as well as tutorials for surgeons and updates on techniques for anaesthetists. Pharmacists helped with ward-based teaching, and attended educational events. One-to-one, 'hands on' teaching was essential, but time-consuming, since it was impossible to spare staff time for group sessions. Personal reflection was encouraged with pain nurses keeping clinical and management work diaries. It proved difficult to influence the formal mechanisms of educational funding.

Both hospitals chose an incremental approach. At the *Horton*, the gynaecology ward (a small ward with good team spirit) was chosen as the place to start before the project moved on to other wards. Patients were involved in reviewing information leaflets. At the *John Radcliffe* the initial focus was in trauma and orthopaedic wards. The project overall was publicised at hospital and ward-based meetings and in the hospital newsletters.

Problems encountered at the *Horton* mainly centred on uncertainty about the hospitals future and staff morale, with managers focusing on survival over service quality issues. There was also significant staff turnover with the pharmacist, business manager and clinical audit adviser leaving as well as general clinical staff shortages. There was a lack of IT skills. Two senior anaesthetists were resistant to the plans and emergency medical overflow delayed the patient audits.

Three types of problems slowed progress at the *John Radcliffe*. First, difficulties with *communications*, for example, ensuring that stakeholders were kept informed of progress – at a time of high staff turnover. There was no mechanisms supporting new staff to learn from previous initiatives. Knowledge of clinical and managerial systems remains mainly in people's heads and is not built into systems of care or institutional procedures. Second, providing *education* to all relevant staff was difficult, especially when it involved releasing groups of nurses from clinical duties. Third, insufficient *nursing resources* meant staff have little capacity for reflecting on new ideas and methods of practice.

Despite the problems, significant improvements were achieved without large financial expenditure – though *a huge investment of time was necessary*: at least half a day a week for one of the local project leaders. In the absence of adequate systems, the main means for maintaining the quality of care relies on repeated education and motivation.

At the *John Radcliffe*, sustaining the changes might necessitate an acute pain service with dedicated nursing and medical sessional time and the development of in-service education and training mechanisms. Trauma ward guidelines could be extended to all surgical wards. For other acute pain areas there should be provision for post-discharge pain management. More might be done on making available more complex techniques (e.g. epidural infusions) and facilities for patients requiring complex forms of pain relief.

At the *Horton*, there is need to maintain daily pain rounds on all surgical wards, the regular update of materials (e.g. guidelines, patients' leaflets). The need for the employment of a third consultant anaesthetist has become clear as well as the need for the post of acute pain nurse to become permanent.

There were some general issues common to both hospitals. The lack of systems of care and insufficient attention to quality issues was exacerbated by a reluctance of influential staff to tackle these problems. There seemed no mechanism for co-ordinating the work of support services such as clinical audit, education and IT. The experience from both hospitals is that under these circumstances clinical staff do not function to the optimum effect. An organised working environment is required in which processes and systems support and enable clinicians to deliver first class care. Clinical governance might offer the prospect of solving some of these dysfunctional problems.

What changed?

A programme of sequential audits was conducted to evaluate this project. This included an initial 'baseline' survey of post-operative patients (September 1996). Baseline information included demographic data, the type and complexity of surgery, the patients' post-operative pain experiences and the pain relieving techniques that were used. A further questionnaire was sent to patients during the week they were sent home from the wards. The questionnaire was designed to elicit patients' pain experience following discharge and the need for medical assistance as a result of pain. Fifteen months later (February 1998) a further group of patients were surveyed to see whether there had been any changes in the quality of acute pain management. The main indicators used to assess the impact of the work were:

1. *Changes in the level of information provision across different staff groups*
2. *Changes in patients perception of pain at rest and pain on movement*
3. *Incidence of nausea and vomiting*
4. *Acceptability of pain treatment compared to actual pain on movement*
5. *A questionnaire sent to patients at home after discharge*

Overall the project has shown that the introduction of a programme of education and clinical guidelines can produce improvements in post-operative pain relief – without the need for expenditure of large sums of money. There was a reduction of pain experienced by patients following surgery and severe post-operative pain was almost eliminated in the second survey. One of the specific recommendations from the project at the John Radcliffe Hospital is the need to address the provision of pain management following discharge from hospital.

The following charts, drawn from the work at the two hospitals, illustrate aspects of the evaluation.

Information provision

Who provided information to patients? (Results from both hospitals)

	Initial survey		Second survey	
Information provider	John Radcliffe	Horton	John Radcliffe	Horton
Ward nurse	22	16	73	9
Surgeon	3	2	15	3
Anaesthetist	27	31	65	59
Others	3	10	1	41

Was information about pain relief given to patients pre-operatively and was this information useful? (Results from the Horton Hospital)

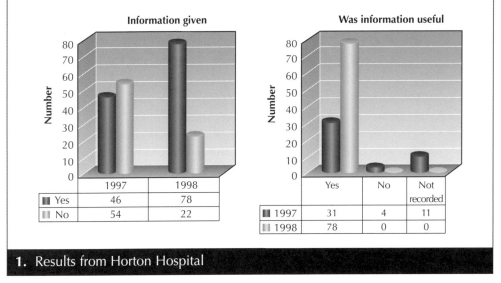

	1997	1998
■ Yes	46	78
▨ No	54	22

	Yes	No	Not recorded
■ 1997	31	4	11
▨ 1998	78	0	0

1. Results from Horton Hospital

Patients' perception of pain (Results from the John Radcliffe Hospital)

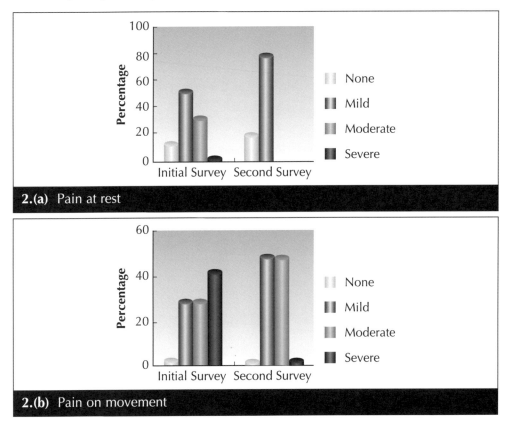

2.(a) Pain at rest

2.(b) Pain on movement

There was an improvement between the two surveys in all aspects of pain.

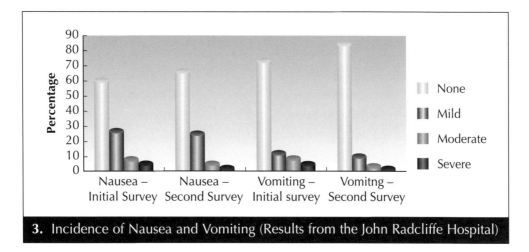

3. Incidence of Nausea and Vomiting (Results from the John Radcliffe Hospital)

Acceptability of pain treatment (Results from the John Radcliffe Hospital)

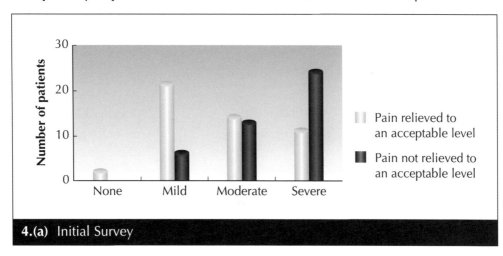

4.(a) Initial Survey

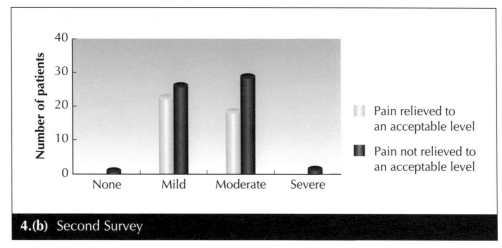

4.(b) Second Survey

Home Questionnaire

Results from the John Radcliffe Hospital

There was little difference between the two surveys. It is a matter of concern that over 50 per cent of the patients experience moderate to severe pain on the day before and on the day of discharge from hospital and 20 per cent still experienced moderate to severe pain up to ten days after leaving hospital.

Appendix

Project leaders and contacts for the 16 PACE projects

The care and treatment of cardiac patients

Lambeth, Southwark and Lewisham and King's Healthcare: cardiac rehabilitation

Project Leader: Dr Brian Fisher, Primary Care Development Practitioner
Project Co-ordinator: Caris Bevan

Contact:
Dr Brian Fisher
Primary Care Development Practitioner
Lambeth, Southwark and Lewisham Health Authority
1 Lower Marsh
LONDON SE1 7NT

Tel: 0171 716 7618; Fax: 0171 716 7018

North Derbyshire: congestive cardiac failure

Project Leader: Dr Carol Singleton, Consultant in Public Health
Project Co-ordinator: Anne Hayes

Contact:
Dr Carol Singleton
Consultant in Public Health
North Derbyshire Health Authority
Scarsdale
Newbold Road
CHESTERFIELD S41 7PF

Tel: 01246 231255; Fax: 01246 206672

South Tyneside: the management of stable angina

Project Leader: Dr John Parr, Consultant Physician

Contact:
Dr John Parr
Consultant Physician
South Tyneside District Hospital
Harton Lane
SOUTH SHIELDS NE34 0PL

Tel: 0191 454 8888

The prevention and management of stroke

Barnet: hypertension in the elderly

Project Leader: Dr Tony Isaacs, Consultant in Clinical Auditing
Project Co-ordinator: Julie Gottlieb

Contact:
Dr Tony Isaacs
Consultant in Clinical Auditing
Barnet Health Authority
Hyde House
The Hyde
Edgware Road
LONDON NW9 6LH

Tel: 0181 201 4700; Fax: 0181 201 4702

Gloucestershire Royal: the management of stroke patients

Project Leader: Janet Duberley, Nurse Executive Director
Project Manager: Bev Williams

Contact:
Bev Williams
PACE Project Manager
Department of Clinical Audit
Gloucestershire Royal NHS Trust
Great Western Road
GLOUCESTER GL1 3NN

Tel: 01452 394869; Fax: 01452 394868

The care and treatment of patients with mental health problems

Wirral: family support in schizophrenia

Project Leader: Nick Morris, Commissioning Manager

Contact:
Mr Nick Morris
Commissioning Manager
Wirral Health
St Catherine's Hospital
Tranmere
BIRKENHEAD L42 0LQ

Tel: 0151 651 0011; Fax: 0151 652 2668

The eradication of *H. pylori* in the management of dyspepsia

Bradford

Project Leader: Dr John Wright, Consultant Epidemiologist
Project Manager: Julie Hughes

Contact:
Julie Hughes
Bradford and Airedale MAAG
New Mill
Victoria Road
Saltaire
SHIPLEY BD18 3LD

Tel: 01274 366234; Fax: 01274 53921
E-mail: julie.hughes@bradford-ha.northy.nhs.uk

Bromley

Project Leader: Steve Dewar, Head of Applied Research Unit
Project Co-ordinator: Jon Pearson

Contact:
Olwen Wade-Jones
Bromley Applied Research Unit
Bromley Hospitals NHS Trust
Farnborough Hospital
Farnborough Common
ORPINGTON BR6 8ND

Tel: 01689 814377
E-mail: aru@direct.co.uk

Walsall

Project Leader: Dr Jeff Norwood, Consultant in Public Health Medicine

Contact:
Dr Jeff Norwood
Consultant in Public Health Medicine
Walsall Health Authority
Lichfield House
27–31 Lichfield House
WALSALL WS1 1TE

Tel: 01922 720255; Fax: 01922 722051

The management of continence

Dudley

Project Manager: Dr Wendy Phillips, Specialist Registrar
Project Co-ordinator: Gill Wellington

Contact:
Gill Wellington
Continence Adviser
Dudley Priority Health NHS Trust
Wordsley Green Health Centre
Wordsley Green
Wordsley
WEST MIDLANDS DY8 5BN

Tel: 01384 457373; Fax: 01384 400217

Wigan and Bolton

Project Leader: Dr Sally Bradley, Consultant in Public Health Medicine
Project Co-ordinator: Rose Moran

Contact:
Dr Sally Bradley
Consultant in Public Health Medicine
Salford and Trafford Health Authority
Peel House
Albert Street
Eccles
MANCHESTER M30 0NJ

Tel: 0161 787 0354; Fax: 0161 787 0237

The care and treatment of patients predominantly in primary care

Dorset: menorrhagia

Project Leader: Dr Vicky Hempsall, Deputy Director of Public Health
Project Manager: Joy Reynolds

Contact:
Sandra Roberts
Clinical Effectiveness Manager
Dorset Health Authority
Victoria House
Princes Road
FERNDOWN BH22 9JR

Tel: 01202 893000

Royal Berkshire: leg ulcers

Project Leader: Chrissie Dunn, Senior Nurse Practice Development
Project Nurse: Trish Powell

Contact:
Chrissy Dunn
Senior Nurse Practice Development
Battle Hospital
Oxford Road
READING RG3 1AG

Tel: 01189 583666; Fax: 01189 636438

Southern Derbyshire: back pain

Project Leader: Dr Steve Whitehead, Director of Public Health
Project Manager: Steve Spear

Contact:
Dr Steve Whitehead
Director of Public Health
Southern Derbyshire Health Authority
Derwent Court
Stuart Street
DERBY DE1 2FZ

Tel: 01332 626300; Fax: 01332 636350

The care of patients in hospital

Chase Farm: Pressure sores

Project Leader: Ms Janice Sigsworth, Director of Nursing
Project Co-ordinator: Julie Baker

Contact:
Julie Baker
Practice Development Facilitator
Old Toronto Ward
Chase Farm Hospital NHS Trust
The Ridgeway
ENFIELD EN2 8JL

Tel: 0181 366 6600

Oxfordshire: Post-operative pain control

Project Leader: Dr Nick Hicks, Consultant Public Health Physician

Contact:
Dr David Mason
Theatres and Anaesthetics Clinical Centre
Oxford Radcliffe NHS Hospital Trust
John Radcliffe Hospital, Level One
Headley Way
OXFORD OX3 9DU

Tel: 01865 222916